Let's heal... xo Kathy Arnos

Walking A Friend Home

A Practical Guide to Consciously Living & Dying

By Kathy Arnos

Foreword by Jeff Kober

ISBN: 978-0-9725783-1-8 — paperback
ISBN: 978-0-9725783-2-5 — e-book

All quotes, excerpts, and stories were reprinted with permission from the authors or representative organizations.

Library of Congress Control Number: 2024906619

Cover design and photos "Into the Light" and "The Veil"
by Kathy Arnos
Author photos by Danielle Arnos
Interior photos by, or the property of Kathy Arnos

Spirit Dance Publishing 爱 A Division of Whole Planet Productions
www.kathyarnos.com

Advance Praise for Walking A Friend Home

"Arnos' words, woven with elegance and warmth, have become a comforting companion, gently guiding me through the complexities of life while providing invaluable insights into understanding and embracing mortality."

Kristofer Updike ~ *Award-winning TV and film producer*

"It is thanks to the commitment to Truth of teachers like Kathy that we can expand into our own lives and deaths to find the purpose we are meant to find so that we, too, may pass on to others the keys to freedom and the willingness to love that we discover for ourselves along the way."

Jeff Kober ~ *Award-winning actor, meditation teacher, and author of Embracing Bliss: 108 Daily Meditations*

"What a breathtakingly beautiful book filled with spiritual, emotional, and actionable guidance to live life fully – in every moment. It gave me a new perspective on the human connection with resilience. Arnos has created a wonderful gift for us all."

Erin Gray ~ *Award-winning actor, speaker, author, and tai chi teacher*

"A powerful read that sparks wonder and tears. The stories strengthen our hope that death is not the end … not by a longshot."

Mimi Kennedy ~ *Award-winning actor and author*

"Walking a Friend Home is a TREASURE! Arnos bridges the process of death in a unique, beautiful, loving way. Each chapter is a glimpse into a greater understanding of this amazing journey of life and death — transforming fears into grace, love, and courage."

Marla Frees ~ *Author of American Psychic, psychic medium, and consciousness coach*

"You do not have to entirely agree with Kathy's philosophy of life, the afterlife, and the space between to receive the gifts this book has to offer. Kathy writes as she lives ... with generosity, kindness, thoughtfulness, and love."

Kay Lenz ~ *Award-winning actor*

"More than words, more than ideas and images … I'm right there in the room with Kathy, her mom, and her dad … Her voice creates a consistency and awareness of things that is not just storytelling but experience sharing."

James Pluta ~ *Award-winning concert film producer*

"It's interesting how all our lives we use the word 'deadline' without hesitation. I have a deadline… you have a deadline. A mystical measure of an ending time for this life as we know it. The brilliance of our creation, our enfoldment, and our participation in life require us to know one day, the deadline is upon us.

There are many teachers who teach us how to grieve after death, yet few true masters who teach us how to grieve death while we are living. Thus, those who grieve death while living are individuals who are totally alive while they are here. Welcome to the "Alive Tribe." Thank you, Kathy Arnos!"

Rev. Temple Hayes ~ *Author of When Did You Die? Eight Steps to Stop Dying Every Day and Start Waking Up*

WAFH is a thoughtful and heartwarming book about a subject that up to now is rarely spoken about yet is an integral part of life — death. Kathy has deftly woven universal teachings and practical wisdom into her personal experiences, sharing the profound sweetness and richness of healing that can take place while navigating this sacred passage home for loved ones and friends.

Rev. Wendy Silvers ~ *Spiritual teacher, speaker, and founder of the Million Mamas Movement*

This book is dedicated to my mother, Laura, and father, Dan …
along with all of the other beloved souls I've had the privilege and
blessing of knowing and supporting in transitioning home who
taught me great lessons about living, loving, and dying —
my treasured teachers.

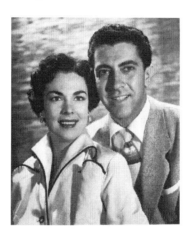

And

In memory of David Bower, my lifelong friend, and soulmate,
whose unconditional love and support are forever
imprinted in my heart!

Disclaimer: The information in this book is intended for reference purposes only, and is not meant to diagnose any condition, or as an endorsement for any entity or organization, product, or prescription for the use of any of the modalities. Even though all of the methods, and products are considered safe, it is hard to predict any one person's response to their use. Always seek the advice of a medical, mental health professional, or legal counsel before starting or using any new form of therapy, and/or engaging in end-of-life planning. The author and publisher disclaim all responsibility for any effects that may occur due to the mention or context in this book.

Reprint Permission Rights

[1] Hanh, T. N. (2011). The Long Road Turns to Joy: A Guide to Walking Meditation. Parallax Press. Quote reprinted in compliance with Parallax Press fair use guidelines parallax.org.

[2] "Osho Zen Tarot ~ The Transcendental Game of Zen. Published 1994 St. Martin's Press. Page 112/Commentary text "Letting Go" reprinted with permission from OSHO International.

[3] Fred Rogers, quote reprinted with permission from Fred Rogers Productions, Licensing Dept.

[4] Brown, B. (2017). Rising Strong: How the Ability to Reset Transforms the Way We Live, Love, Parent, and Lead. Random House. Quote reprinted in compliance with BrenéBrown.com permission guidelines.

[5] Ostaseski, F. (2017) The Five Invitations: Discovering What Death Can Teach Us About Living Fully. New York: Flatiron Books. Quote reprinted with permission from the author.

TABLE OF CONTENTS

FOREWORD BY JEFF KOBER

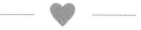

All of life is but a stepping toward death.

If you ever want to stop a conversation, mentioning the above is almost guaranteed to do so — especially in Western culture, in which virtually no one likes to talk about it or be reminded of the certainty of death.

We tend to fear death and see it as an ending, nothingness, or a vague notion of perfection that we will find in "heaven" if we play our cards right.

Thankfully, there is a different way of looking at things.

In the East, death is not seen as the opposite of life but rather as a part of life, valued as something sacred and profound — without which life could not exist. It is as basic and essential as birth, hunger, thirst, and procreation. The certainty of death allows us to value life in a way that is true and real rather than as a series of acquisitions. Knowing that all shall pass causes us to insist on finding meaning and value in the unseen.

I met Kathy Arnos in 2010; like me, she was looking for answers to these big questions. A mutual friend suggested she learn Vedic meditation, which I teach, and from that day to this, we've shared the path toward wholeness.

We, humans, are driven by our needs. The need to survive, reproduce, find our tribe, and seek comfort. All of us discover at some point that there is no arrangement or amount of these qualities in a life that offers us peace. There is always something missing.

All spiritual paths speak of this missing thing: that beneath the ever-changing nature of life, there is a place of Truth — "truth" in the sense that it's always there, always the same, regardless of whatever might be happening on the surface of things. No matter how furious the storm is on the surface of the ocean, in the depths, we will find a place of peace and calm and the sense that things are okay. When we find this place within, often found via meditation (or other spiritual practices), our lives change.

To have peace within and always available is more than enough for some people. For others, the questioning continues. Kathy is one of those who, in finding wholeness in life, also found that this wholeness is just the beginning — a starting point for more questions about life itself, which lead inevitably to the subject of this book: Death and its place in life, within our own life and of those we love.

Kathy is a healer and a teacher. She has spent her time helping others navigate life, death, and things in between in a meaningful fashion. And like all dedicated teachers, Kathy has used her own life as a laboratory to see what works and what doesn't — learning on the job, as it were, how to free ourselves from fear and how to come out of ignorance and into acceptance of life and the way it happens, rather than the way we think it should be happening. She has learned how to offer herself an experience of life that is grand enough to encompass even death without losing the sense of wonder and the opportunity for joy that life truly is.

Kathy has learned and lived these truths and embodied them so that she might offer them to others with kindness, compassion, vulnerability, and love. In other words, she teaches as she lives and teaches what she lives. The resonance of this authenticity and sincerity invites you to open up in kind and see your own path forward, your own version of the lived wisdom this book offers.

Without the certainty of death, life has no meaning. Without the need and the opportunity to learn, life has no purpose. Without the wise guidance of those who have gone before, we might spend decades, even lifetimes, walking in circles and wondering why we never arrive anywhere.

It is thanks to the commitment to Truth of teachers like Kathy that we ourselves can expand into our own lives and deaths to find the purpose we are meant to find so that we, too, may pass on to others the keys to freedom and the willingness to love that we discover for ourselves along the way.

Jeff Kober, actor, meditation teacher,
author of Embracing Bliss and host
of the Embracing Bliss podcast

INTRODUCTION

Death is awkward, so let's talk about it with love, humor, and gratitude! What if you could learn how to live life intentionally, totally awake and aware — and die consciously, with a full heart, grace, dignity, connection, and feeling complete?

Walking a Friend Home: A Practical Guide to Consciously Living & Dying invites you to move from the intellectual mind into the spirit of the heart and explore your human vulnerability to best prepare for death, one of life's most inevitable moments.

How Do We Navigate This Complex Journey of Life and Death?

Walking A Friend Home is a step-by-step guide that combines practical information with personal stories about the intimacy of relationships. It blends spiritual, holistic, and conventional methods to create a memorable last chapter for everyone through awareness, conversation, planning, and cultivating deeper connections.

The book answers fundamental questions (you might be afraid to ask) and provides tools, techniques, and resources to:

- Overcome your fears and foster honest communication
- Practice acts of service, self-care, and mindfulness
- Efficiently plan for all phases — emotionally, physically, logistically, and spiritually
- Move beyond past resentments and find forgiveness, compassion, and unconditional love
- Gently surf the ocean waves of grief

- Learn how to be with your loved one in a new way after they are physically gone

We will all experience the loss of a loved one at some point. Sadly, many of us will walk the path of transition on our own and die alone with no emotional, spiritual, or physical support from those we love or logistical preparation to meet this end-of-life experience.

The reason for this is simple — broaching the subject of death is extremely uncomfortable! Despite its certainty, the thought of death or having a conversation about it is so terrifying that some people would rather die alone than discuss it. This book guides you to move through your fear and begin a dialog with those you care about. When you permit yourself to have honest conversations about death, you'll experience a greater sense of belonging and connection throughout your life and die with a feeling of completion. (See Chapter 3, "Making Friends with Death,".)

As a holistic practitioner and health writer, I have spent decades teaching people about consciously living with intention. I have done so in various ways: in my private practice, as a journalist and author, through live events, workshops, classes, and on national radio and television.

Throughout my career, I have utilized the knowledge gained through my studies with inspirational teachers, doctors, and others who have helped me formulate my truth. Not everyone will share this truth. This book reflects my thoughts and beliefs about birth, life, death, and the afterlife — the entire cycle of life.

It's odd to think that three words — birth, life, and death — describe the only certainties in our existence. These three words look simple and finite when you see them on paper. But when experienced, these life stages are complex and multi-layered — each beckoning us to stay present and mindful throughout.

Unfortunately, many of us miss out on the beauty of the different aspects of each phase because we're stuck in our past hurts and future projections, unable to connect to the present moment without fear of the unknown. We get caught up in our distracted, busy lifestyles, distorted emotional thinking, flawed reasoning, or generational beliefs, which rob us of each phase's gifts.

And even though death comes at the end of life, from the time we are born, we are preparing for it — whether we know it or not. The irony of this is we can't consciously prepare for death until we can talk about it and have a clearer understanding of what death means to us, and about the process of dying itself.

Early Education and Conversations are the Best Paths to Understanding Death

One element often overlooked as we approach death is that human beings are social creatures that need love, support, and nurturing to thrive and feel connected. Like the other phases of life, I believe we should also take the last part of our journey — aging, illness, and transition — together. For me, love, considered one of the most powerful energy sources in the world, is part of this connection. In caring for my family, I've discovered that this exchange of energy can transform even the most difficult relationships.

The actual act of dying is a dance with and into different dimensions through an integration process enhanced by this love and care of others. Without this emotional completion, those dying and those who remain are left with a deprivation of spirit.

I have personally experienced death through both the silence of emotional dispossession and by being part of someone's supportive process. My mother died when I was eleven years old without talking to me about her illness or preparing me for her death. This act of avoidance and denial, although unconscious, left me feeling emotionally and physically alone, confused, and traumatized. Thankfully, the flipside to that came decades later when my father was diagnosed with terminal cancer, and he and I began a conversation and journey together that would completely change my thoughts and views about living and dying.

That experience was an incredible gift (for both of us) and taught me great lessons about the depths of relationships, communication, and the interconnectedness of all things in life — especially unconditional love. It opened my heart and was the beginning of many unexpected opportunities for me to walk others home in years to come.

Understanding the Intimacy of Relationships Through Acts of Service

When I began sharing stories about being around loved ones in transition, people — some of them strangers — would thank me. I discovered that many of them had never openly discussed death with anyone other than me before, yet, they were curious and willing to listen, ask questions, and learn about the process.

In those moments, I realized how these conversations could gently open a door and make space for people to think and talk about this intimidating, taboo subject. It offered them a unique way to unwrap their inner fears and shift their perspective of the dying process, even if ever so slightly, and begin to release their negative thoughts. I now understand how critical this intimate conversation is to ultimately live life more fully. Part of being alive is being aware of our death.

As I mentioned earlier, throughout this book, you will find a variety of personal stories that I have written, along with some anecdotes by dear friends willing to share their stories.

All of the narrations speak to the intimacy of relationships, unconditional love, compassion, forgiveness, healing, and gratitude — how to find, feel, give, and receive it through acts of kindness and being present for those we love.

The first six vignettes, which you'll find in between the book's early chapters, introduce my biological and extended family. They were my earliest and most significant teachers who showed me the value of walking a friend or loved one home. These stories give you a glimpse into the history of each relationship so you can fully appreciate the dynamics and the gifts that came with being of service to them in the end.

The next series of vignettes between Chapters 6 through 10 are about walking some of my other friends home. These experiences offered me different perspectives on witnessing and supporting people through their process without the emotional family enmeshment. Each one surprised me in ways that revealed something new about telepathically communicating with those in transition, what people wait for, the spirit beings that come to greet us, the confusion that can take place for an integrating soul, and how the karmic plan takes care of divine timing so beautifully.

The healing I witnessed and received by being part of all these experiences (and others) was an exchange of energy that has to be lived to be appreciated. It opened the door to an essence of this rare form of intimacy and love that I never knew existed, and it allowed me to discover my unconditional self.

My wish in sharing these stories is that they help inspire you to connect with someone you love while they are still alive, whether you have had a loving relationship with that person or a challenging one, and begin the conversation. Everyone deserves to be loved and — when possible — walked home with dignity.

All of the stories presented in this book are the respective person's or my recollections and interpretation of the experience or event. Not everyone will see or remember them in the same way. When you can find the courage to participate in helping somebody transition home, it's an extraordinary experience that cannot fully be put into words but rather a richness of emotion that is quite remarkable.

I invite you to take the journey with me as I share new concepts for reflection that stretch the imagination about where we come from, where we might go in the end, and how to be with our loved ones in a new way when they are physically gone. I have learned much about the importance of living and dying well and how to prepare emotionally, physically, logistically, and spiritually for this rite of passage. I look forward to helping you do the same — like walking a friend home at the end of a long day — *a day that will change your life forever.*

CHAPTER 1

A BIT OF HISTORY: AN AWARENESS
OF DIMENSIONAL SIGHT

Understanding & Working with Energy

As a child, I remember having a relationship with the spirit world, energetic resonance, and the earthly dimension. I was vibrationally sensitive, which meant I could see in the dark and feel people's energy fields. When I looked at the sky or the air in a room, I could see the movement of electricity and energy particles. Sometimes, this moving matter was associated with different colors. I also spent a lot of time alone playing and communicating with spirit beings, or what some might consider imaginary friends, never questioning their energy.

I assumed other kids had similar experiences, but I later realized that most didn't or hadn't yet learned how to recognize and interact with this invisible force.

As I grew older, my fascination with these unexplainable experiences grew. In my teens, I also realized I had a unique sense of "knowing." Not omniscience, but more like an inner voice that told me things I ordinarily might not be aware of — a form of clairvoyance. Often, when someone asked me a question, a response would flow out of my mouth as if someone were feeding me the information. What came through me intuitively and naturally was inevitably what that person needed to hear.

My first memory of communicating with someone I knew in the spirit world came after my mother died when I was eleven. She began interacting with me every year on New Year's Day — the last time I saw her just before she passed away. Initially, this annual experience was more overt. For example, when I was in my late teens, I was kneeling in my closet, and something fell from the top shelf, brushing the back of my head. My friend, who was sitting across the room, asked, "What was that?" When I turned around, there was a picture on the floor behind me of my mother and me at a birthday party that I had never seen before. As time passed, her communication shifted and became more sensory, like wind or sound-oriented, almost like hearing a voice — not necessarily hers, but rather an audio frequency transmission of some kind.

My dreams (past and present) also often contain messages from or about people on the other side for their loved ones, occasionally even offering me a full conversation with them. When I wake up after having one of these dreams, no matter how hard I try to dismiss the message as insignificant, I know I must share it.

Years ago, I was cleaning my desktop and found a sticky note I had forgotten about with a message for one of my friends that included several numbers. I had received it in a dream a few weeks earlier, around Thanksgiving. I'm never sure what numbers mean — it could be a date, monetary amount, or lock combination — but I always make a note of them.

This particular message was from my friend's beloved partner of 20 years, who had unexpectedly passed away a few years before without appropriately providing for her future. This mistake prompted years of legal issues between her and his family. It read,

"I am so sorry! I love you," and then I was shown the numbers. I hadn't spoken to my friend in months, but when I came across the Post-it note, I texted her the message. She wasn't surprised and shared that she had felt his presence strongly around that time. After reflecting on the numbers, she later texted me and said when she separated the numbers, she realized they were the date he died. I felt he included those numbers to prove that his amends and expression of love were truly a communication from him.

Like with all things in life, the evolution of my interdimensional skills has shifted and changed over the years. Being with my father in his final weeks was especially insightful. He was a great teacher and willing to share everything he was experiencing with me. I became the listener, the student. Our relationship during this time opened the door to another realm of discovery — a deeper connection with my intuition and the spirit world.

The fruits of this instructive relationship were apparent even before my dad passed away. For example, when I invited my dad's sister Ida to say goodbye to him, I was saddened to hear she wouldn't be able to visit for a couple of weeks and was skeptical he would last that long. To my surprise, when I asked my father, he got excited and, after a moment of reflection, said yes, he would be there.

True to his word, my dad took his last breath the day after Ida went home.

That experience showed me that those in transition often can wait for something to feel complete. This happened again with my stepmother and has continued with those I've assisted ever since. I can tune into their souls and ask them what they're waiting for — even if they aren't audible or conscious — to facilitate their needs being met. I write about this completion phenomenon in all of my stories. In each case, it is different and, at times, very surprising as to what they are waiting for to find completion.

I also discovered that in addition to waiting for something, people also begin a dance with — and between — the two worlds as they integrate with the other side. I've noticed that two interesting things take place simultaneously:

- The (still) living are drawn to energetically sensitive people (like myself) who are attuned to this mixed realm experience — physical and ethereal.
- Spirit beings from the other side (family, friends, and even strangers) usually come to greet them and have conversations with them in preparation for their last breath and transition.

Many people don't always understand what is happening when their loved one moves into a liminal state and starts interacting with those on the other side. They dismiss the conversations or sightings as delusional or a hallucination, which I believe is not the case.

With that thought in mind, the next time someone you know is approaching their final weeks or days and is having random conversations with their invisible friends, try to sit and listen with an open mind and acknowledge their experience. You might just be witnessing a rare interdimensional exchange. This allows you to be part of the conversation with their unique support team (the spirit beings), who have come to make their journey through transition easier and feel a little safer.

Our time and ability to listen are two valuable gifts we can give someone. I have found that by doing so, I have developed a deeper understanding and appreciation for these moving souls' remarkable journey going home … a gift I would like to share with you through my stories and experiences.

MY MOTHER: SAYING GOODBYE

Vignette One

♥

My mother was a single, hard-working woman. She was a make-up artist in the entertainment industry, which made for a colorful life with creative characters and wild parties. In the '60s, she developed one of the first consumer make-up kits to hit the market. Before meeting my dad, she was a dancer in USO shows for the military, danced on stage in Vegas, and eventually went on to television. Needless to say, my life was anything but normal.

Mom spent most of her time away from home at the studios working with actresses, designers, and models as she tried to juggle the logistics of being a single mom and raising me. Consequently, there wasn't much time for us.

Since my mother was rarely home before dinner or bedtime, I only had a few fond memories of her and me alone — cooking clam sauce spaghetti late at night, watching The *Wizard of Oz* together, or snuggling in bed first thing in the morning. I cherished those rare intimate mother-daughter moments of connection, something I so desperately craved.

My parents divorced when I was two, and Mom and I lived in an upscale neighborhood of the Santa Monica Mountains in a somewhat neglected and chaotic household along with my 83-year-old recently widowed grandmother, another single working mom named Arlie, who ran a modeling agency, and her 18-month-old son.

My father had pretty much been absent in my life up to this stage, mainly because of his addictions — drugs and alcohol — and bad choices that landed him in trouble. When I got older, my father used to say one of his biggest regrets was how neglected I was as a child. More about him later.

The Mystery

In early November 1966, I left home rushing to catch the school bus like I did every morning. Honestly, I don't remember if I saw my mom or even said goodbye that day. She hadn't been feeling well for over a year, so it wasn't unusual for her to sleep in and for us not to connect in the morning. I was 11, and like most preteens, I lived in my self-absorbed world.

My mother wasn't there when I got home from school that day. My grandmother said some friends had come by to pick her up, and she didn't know where they were going or when they would return. It seemed odd, but I didn't think anything more about it until bedtime, when I still hadn't heard from her. I assumed I'd see her before school; however, her bed was empty the following morning.

Over the next 24 hours, I became increasingly worried because it was so out of character for my mom not to check in with me. In the past, if she was going to be late or stay away overnight, she either called or left me a note; this time, there was nothing.

When I asked Arlie about her sudden disappearance, she said that my mother would be away working on a special project for a few weeks. When I said I wanted to speak to her, Arlie gave me a phone number to reach her in the afternoon after school. At that age, I was very literal and thought that was the only time slot I could call her. The next day, when I called the number, a woman answered and said she would see if my mother was available. I waited three or four minutes — an eternity to my anxious mind — before someone picked up the extension phone. The slurred, thick voice on the other end was hard to understand, and it took me a minute to realize it was my mother. When I asked her if she had been sleeping, she said yes and asked if we could talk tomorrow.

After that, my mother was rarely available when I called, and the few times we did speak, our communication was always the same and very one-way— "Hi, Mom, I miss you. When will you be home? I can't understand you." Something was obviously wrong, but I didn't know what to do.

In the '60s, no one ever discussed feelings or critical issues with children like divorce, illness, or death. The truth was that my mother had cancer, and her collective group of friends had decided it was best not to tell me. Consequently, I was left in the dark, feeling sad, scared, and abandoned. I missed my mother terribly.

Several weeks passed, and still, no one spoke about her whereabouts or when she might return. We had moved up into the canyon a few years earlier, leaving our close friends behind, so I was extremely lonely. By now, it was December, and Christmas was fast approaching. Christmas was one of my favorite holidays because my mom always ensured Santa brought me new clothes, which was a real treat for me instead of hand-me-downs. It was also a time for getting together with my mom's best friend Gloria, a writer and one of Hollywood's young starlets who found her inspiration in a bottle, and her daughter Lexy, who was (and still is) one of my closest friends.

My mom had never missed a Christmas, and I could feel my disappointment growing around not seeing her or my friends. Since Arlie was my only connection to my mom, I continued to pester her for answers about when I'd see or talk to her again, but her response was always the same: "Hopefully soon."

Christmas Day

Three days before Christmas, my stepmother, Rose, phoned and told me that my mother was in the hospital. She said she would pick me up on Christmas day to take me to see her and that I should wear a dress and be ready by noon. Her call was confusing because I thought my mom was away working on a project, so I didn't understand why she was suddenly in the hospital.

In any event, I was grateful I would get to see her but resentful that I had to wear a dress to do it. I hated wearing dresses because I was overweight, and they were uncomfortable. I also associated them with going to school, which triggered additional anxiety because I struggled with an undiagnosed learning disability. The whole situation was upsetting and humiliating. Still, I pushed past my feelings, squeezed into my corduroy jumper, and was ready on time. After all, I was going to see my mom!

My father had a history of being unreliable (again, more on that later), so it was no surprise that Rose came alone to pick me up that day. I don't remember much about the drive other than the awkward silence I felt being with this woman I didn't know or like very much. Rose was not warm and fuzzy or even very approachable. She criticized me (well, more accurately, my parents' neglect of me), which made me feel small and never good enough. That said, she had some degree of compassion as she at least took an interest in my needs being met. Rose was the responsible one and even more annoying, perfect in her appearance. In contrast, I struggled with my unkempt clothes and body image.

I had a lot of questions about why my mom was in the hospital — and about my mom and dad's absences in general — but I certainly didn't feel comfortable asking Rose about either one. Despite all of my confusion, I was grateful and excited that I would get to see my mom after what seemed like an eternity.

After an endless ride through parts of the city I had never seen before, we finally arrived at an old flat building that looked more like a motel than a hospital. Rose was in a hurry and verbally hustled me along as she marched ahead of me across the parking lot. "What's wrong with you, can't you go any faster?" and "Don't you want to see your mother?"

Once inside, I felt apprehensive and out of place as the staff tried to find a discreet area for me to sit in. Eventually, a nurse brought me a rickety folding chair and placed it outside my mother's shared room in a bright fluorescent-lit hallway. I had to take shallow breaths to avoid the stench of chemicals and illness that permeated the building. My heart felt like it would burst through my tight jumper, and it took everything I had not to run out of the nearby emergency exit.

Several of my mother's close friends, including Gloria, came and went from the room, whispering as they briefly acknowledged my presence. Whatever was happening in that room was a mystery, so I remained in my designated seat, motionless like a soldier waiting in a foxhole. Suddenly, there was a lot of commotion inside the room. Alarms rang, and the door swung open and slammed shut. The medical staff ran in and out like they were under siege.

A nurse grabbed hold of the chair and ejected me to make way for a crash cart whizzing by full of emergency equipment. My heart jumped into my throat as I tried to get a glimpse of my mother.

Before I could see her, the same nurse motioned for me to take a seat again as she slammed the door shut. Someone had moved my chair across the hall, so I dutifully sat back down.

Once things settled down, my stepmother reappeared for a minute to tell me I couldn't see my mother. Her normally coiffed hair was amiss, and she was visually shaken. After she rushed back into the room, I felt my throat constricting as the sting of hot tears of disappointment ran down my cheeks. I didn't know what to do, so I closed my eyes tightly. I figured if I couldn't see anyone, I could pretend I was invisible … and silently drift away from this awful nightmare.

A few minutes later, with my eyes still closed, I heard someone awkwardly shuffling around me in the hallway. When I opened my eyes, Rose and Gloria stood before me, holding a wrapped gift. At first, I was so lost in my fear that all I could see were their mouths moving without sound. They appeared to be talking to me, but I couldn't hear their voices. I was promptly jolted back into my body when Rose blurted out, "Just give it to her."

Gloria handed me the gift and said it was from my mother. I wasn't sure what to say or do. I thought I was going to throw up. I had to dig deep to find the courage to stay strong and composed. I tried to hide my tears, but they just kept flowing, and even worse, I was now the center of attention when all I wanted to do was run and hide.

"Open it," they insisted through their quivering voices and bloodshot eyes. "Aren't you going to open it?"

My inner voice screamed, *"I don't want whatever is in the box. I want to see my mother! And if I can't do that, I just want to curl up and disappear."*

I extended my hands, accepted the gift, and opened it to appease them. I even managed to get out a small grunt of gratitude, as it was the gift that, just days before, I had so desperately wanted more than anything in the world (besides seeing my mother) — a Polaroid Swinger camera. It was a bittersweet moment for me.

Shortly afterward, Rose ushered me out of the hospital and drove me home again in silence. There was no conversation about what had happened or acknowledgment of my mom's cancer or my fear. I felt so alone and lost.

When Arlie came home that night, she asked if I had seen my mom. All I could do was shake my head no as I tried to hold back my tears again. Even though Arlie was the one person I trusted, I still felt unsafe expressing my sadness because no one had ever told me that having feelings or expressing them was normal. I will never forget the compassionate look on her face when she saw the pain that I was in.

New Year's Eve

A week passed, and it was now New Year's Eve but still no word about my mother's hospital stay or her health. That night Arlie, my best friend, Pam, Grandma, and I all hung out and watched television and played games. The night's activities were a good distraction, but in the morning, I again asked Arlie when I could speak to or see my mother. She just looked at me with sadness in her eyes and said, "Hopefully soon."

After dinner, Arlie came into the room where Pam and I were playing with her son and said, "Get your jackets, kids. We're going out to run an errand." This request was highly unusual as we lived at the top of a canyon where people didn't go out much at night, especially with a young toddler. Once we were in the car, my curiosity took hold, and I piped up, "Where are we going?" Arlie finally replied that we were going to see my mom.

I was instantly filled with both panic and enthusiasm. Fear, because of the disappointment I had experienced one week earlier, and excitement at the thought of actually seeing my mom this time. The difference was that I was with the two people I knew and trusted most, so I felt a sense of safety.

This ride was much shorter and in a different direction than where I was taken on Christmas Day. We arrived at a small one-story building in Sherman Oaks with an empty parking lot — a very different scenario than the week before. We entered a dimly lit lobby with lots of green plants, a small water fountain, and soft music playing. It was very peaceful and serene.

Saying Goodbye

A woman with a gentle voice was expecting us and took Arlie to see my mother first while we waited in the reception area. Arlie was gone for quite a while, and when she returned, she was crying. I felt a surge of anxiety and disappointment. It was the same sick feeling I had experienced the week before. Maybe I wasn't going to see my mother after all?

However, that was not the case. I followed Arlie into the hallway even though my legs were trembling with fear and resistance, while Pam stayed in the lobby with her son. She could see I was visibly scared and reached for my hand. I wrapped both of my hands around hers as we entered the room. It was dark, and I could only see a dim light coming from behind the privacy curtain. I was afraid of the dark and what might be in this cave-like room. In my world, darkness was where uncertainty lived.

As we moved further into the room, Arlie wriggled out of my grip. Without the reassuring warmth of her hand, I felt impossibly vulnerable and scared.

Arlie whispered to my mom, "Laura, I brought you a surprise. I brought your daughter Kathy to see you. You remember Kathy, don't you?"

Her words and behavior made me even more anxious. *Why wouldn't my mother remember me?*

I had never gone more than a few days without seeing my mother before, so I was a little nervous she might look different. However, as I came around the curtain, nothing could have prepared me for what I saw. The woman buried in the sheets was an unrecognizable, emaciated, gray-haired woman who couldn't have weighed more than 60 pounds. Arlie continued to speak to my mother in a soft voice, gently reminding her several more times that I was her daughter.

Eventually, my mom began moving, using every ounce of strength to navigate the covers and turn her frail body towards us. Once Arlie saw that she was responsive to our presence, she said she would leave so we could have some private time together. I was terrified of being left alone with this sickly-looking stranger. *Who was this woman? How could this be my mother?* I had only known my mother as a vibrant, beautiful, full-figured woman with a spirited personality who could've been Elizabeth Taylor's sister. That was not the woman who was lying in the bed before me.

I had never been around extreme illness or seen such a devastating transformation in a human being. Confused and frightened, I didn't know what to say or do. With trepidation, I slowly approached the side of the bed to get a closer look. I kept trying to make eye contact, but she was having trouble keeping her eyes open.

I eventually mustered up enough courage to speak and said, "You don't look like my mommy. Are you, my mommy?"

Once she heard my voice, something magical happened; she opened her eyes and looked directly into mine. Too weak to speak, she tried to acknowledge my presence and respond to my question with her eyes.

I repeated, "Are you, my mommy?"

She slowly moved her fingers from under the covers towards me to hold my hand. By then, I was crying as we connected through our hearts and eyes — soul to soul — mother to daughter.

I became so overwhelmed with emotion I could barely speak. I told my mother how much I missed and loved her as I gasped for breath through my quivering voice and tears. I kept repeating my feelings over and over. After a few minutes, there was nothing left to say except goodbye.

I leaned over and kissed her head, saying one last time, "I love you," and "Goodbye." She closed her eyes and seemed to be at peace with our experience. I watched her for another minute as I tried to contain my uncontrollable feelings of sadness before leaving the room.
As we left the hospital that night, I remember the awkwardness of my tears and immense confusion and grief as I tried to understand what had just happened. The wave of emotions that filled my heart and spirit that night was indescribable. The impact of the experience was so devastatingly painful that I shut down inside emotionally to survive.

That was the last time I saw my mother. She died a few hours after our visit, a little after midnight. I know now that she had waited for me to say goodbye so she could have a sense of completion. Our journey together in this lifetime was now finished.

Waiting for Completion

Over the years of working with those preparing for death, I have learned when people have a terminal illness, they usually wait for one particular thing to happen to feel complete before making their transition. That one thing could be a relative or friend to visit or an action to take place. Whatever it is, it gives them a sense of completion so they can move on.

Reflecting on my own experience, I know today that my mother waited for someone to have the courage to bring me to her bedside to say goodbye. That someone was Arlie — that special angel brave enough to give my mother and me an invaluable gift I will always remember with the deepest gratitude.

Thanking Arlie

When I started writing this book, I realized how brave Arlie was to have gone against everyone's wishes by taking me to see my mother that night. She allowed her heart to guide her to do what was right for her dear friend Laura and her daughter (me). While I hadn't spoken to Arlie in years, I knew I needed to call her and thank her for the gift she had given us both.

Arlie was then in her eighties and living in the downstairs unit of her son Stephen's house in Utah. I got so excited when I heard her voice, but as we spoke, I quickly realized she had no idea who I was. Given the circumstances, I wasn't sure whether or not she would remember her courageous actions all those years ago.

After further assessing the situation, I decided to tell her why I was calling. She listened intently and then began to cry. She remembered what she had done and could understand and appreciate my infinite gratitude. She said my call was something she would cherish forever.

When I spoke to her son Stephen later that afternoon, he confirmed my suspicion that Arlie had been diagnosed with Alzheimer's. He also said despite her Alzheimer's, whatever I had told her made her very happy, and she wouldn't stop talking about me the rest of the afternoon. She even asked to see my picture and, when she saw it, said, "I remember." I am so grateful that she remembered what had happened!

Arlie passed away a few weeks later with her son and his partner by her side in a loving and supportive environment.

In Reflection

As I mentioned earlier, I believe things happen for a reason and that my mother's choice not to tell me that she had cancer helped shape me into the woman I am today. However, as a mother myself, I cannot imagine not telling my daughter the truth. I sometimes wonder what our time together might have been like in that last phase had we been given the opportunity to take that journey together. While that will forever remain a mystery, I am truly grateful that today I have compassion and forgiveness in my heart surrounding my mother's illness and death.

The main thing I've learned from this childhood experience is how important honesty and communication with our loved ones are during life's events. Hiding the reality of illness or the process of dying only robs people of the support and companionship needed during this critical time. Opening yourself to these experiences has the potential to enhance and heal relationships. Ultimately, intimacy and unconditional love result when we are present for life and death's lessons — a journey that I believe we are here to take together.

CHAPTER 2

MEDITATION: FINDING STILLNESS IN LIFE TO PREPARE FOR DEATH

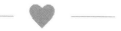

"When we are mindful, deeply in touch with the present moment, our understanding of what is going on deepens, and we begin to be filled with acceptance, joy, peace, and love." ~ Thich Nhat Hanh[1]

Learning About Death with Meditation

If you are new to meditation or uncomfortable with the subject of death, you are probably wondering what these two things have in common. This chapter is about my journey to find that answer.

Meditation is an ancient technique used to redirect the mind from the constant stress and distractions of the external world (while fully awake) to an internal state of calm and relaxation. When we meditate, several spiritual, neurological, and biochemical things occur in the brain and body, including an increase in neurotransmitters and hormones. Countless studies have shown that meditation actually rewires brain circuits that boost mind and body health.

---

[1] Hanh, T. N. (2011). The Long Road Turns to Joy: A Guide to Walking Meditation. Parallax Press. Quote reprinted in compliance with Parallax Press fair use guidelines parallax.org.go

Most people live daily with some degree of emotional or physical stress, whether they are aware of it or not. This type of internal imbalance isn't sustainable for one's optimal health or happiness. Meditation can be instrumental in teaching us how to manage our stress and anxiety levels. It can enhance our self-awareness to live with presence and help us process and release fears, including those about mortality.

Back in the 1990s, my definition of meditation was plain and simple — it was a mind-centering exercise I practiced while doing other things — working in the garden, swimming laps, shoveling horse manure, hiking, or during those few moments just before I fell asleep. It was a time when I reflected on my thoughts, prayed, and reasoned things out. This method served me well.

Several of my friends practiced more formal styles of meditation, but these never appealed to me. I wasn't comfortable kneeling or sitting silently on the floor cross-legged for long periods. It never occurred to me that these other techniques might offer additional emotional, neurological, or spiritual benefits.

It wasn't until 2010, when I met Jeff Kober, a meditation teacher, that I began to explore a more dedicated practice of quietly being with myself — with no distractions. Jeff introduced me to a gentle way of meditating in the Vedic tradition: sitting in a chair (or floor with back support), and effortlessly repeating a mantra to transcend my thoughts for 20 minutes twice daily.

A mantra is a Sanskrit word, phrase, or sound used to "free the mind" (*manas* meaning mind; *trayate* meaning freedom). Depending on your spiritual practice, there are several types of mantras you can use (i.e., healing, affirmation, and devotional). In the Vedic tradition, the type of mantra used is "bija" or seed Mantra. Its purpose is to settle the mind into a more relaxed state of awareness or consciousness — a place of inner coherence, where nothing needs to change for everything to be OK.

If you haven't yet explored the world of meditation, there are various approaches to consider. The process can be as simple as doing a five-minute guided meditation using an app, engaging in intentional chanting, or using a mantra during silent meditation, such as in the Vedic tradition.

There are many choices; finding what's right for you is an individual quest. I found the Vedic tradition to be the most comfortable and easiest form to implement into my daily routine, and it is something I could do anytime or anywhere (and without electronics).

Studies have shown that the profound rest achieved during 20 minutes of meditation can generally be as relaxing and restorative as sleep. This does not mean meditation can replace sleep, but it does allow the nervous system to decompress and relax more deeply than when you are sleeping. You let go of the internal stresses that have accumulated over time — a day, a week, or over a lifetime. By meditating, you learn how to center yourself, let go of habituated stress responses, self-regulate emotional triggers, and develop overall healthier patterns of self-care.

Once I began to meditate regularly, several things happened. I had more energy, clarity, focus, patience, and creative productivity. I also became more conscious of my breathing patterns and engaged with my five senses — both in an awake state and during meditation. This heightened sensory awareness seemed to distract the mind's chatter and give my nervous system time to rest and reset. I spent more time in the present moment experiencing these sensations rather than focusing on my past or projecting into the future.

I found that when I could surrender my thoughts, even if only for a few minutes during my 20-minute meditation (or during my day), a sweet moment of suspension — or transcendence — occurred. I had only experienced this sense of inner peace and trust a few other times before I started intentionally meditating.

One example was when I was snorkeling off Molokai in Hawaii and noticed a shark swimming about 25 feet below me. At first, I was scared, but after assessing that it had no interest in me, a deep feeling of connectedness came over me. It was as if my fear of nature's dangers had disappeared in that split second, leaving behind a feeling of oneness with the entire ocean. My heart and mind merged as my consciousness shifted from intellect to spirit. It was a moment of being in faith that I will never forget.

The logistics of meditating may sound simple, but the discipline itself of making time to actually sit down every day and do it isn't as easy as it sounds. However, the benefits are worth it. The more I meditated, the more these moments of spiritual connection and sense of well-being grew in frequency. Eventually, they began to link together, providing me with an emotional balance that overflowed into my daily life.

As my practice evolved, I learned that the pulse of my heart — considered the seat of the soul — and my breath truly power everything. The heart is the first organ to develop in the body. It consists of approximately 40,000 neurons that create a "little brain" or "intrinsic cardiac nervous system," which continuously sends different signals to the brain. It is well documented that this heart-brain coherence significantly affects the brain's ability to manage trauma and stress. The HeartMath Institute has wonderful readings in this area. Writer and mythologist Joseph Campbell also speaks of this heart-mind connection and coherence with nature in his book, *The Power of Myth*.

That said, you don't have to consciously attain this heart-mind connection or find quietude to benefit from meditating or to be of service to someone in transition. Nor is there a goal in meditation other than making a commitment to yourself to do it consistently once or twice a day.

> *Buddha was asked, "What have you gained from meditation?*
> *He replied, "Nothing!"*
> *However, Buddha said, "Let me tell you what I lost:*
> *Anger, anxiety, depression, insecurity, fear of old age and death."*
> *~ Author Unknown*

A Meditative Path to a Peaceful Death

Another benefit I gained from my practice was I developed a relationship with the mystery of "silence" and found a place where my buried memories lived. I began unearthing them one by one as I healed the old wounds. These feelings can be uncomfortable, but my connection to them has changed over time, and I respond to them differently.

I learned how to process stored trauma by experiencing the emotions associated with the memory as a thought rather than being a victim of the incident, which could then be released. My negative feelings and beliefs that had once triggered anxiety, resentment, fear, mistrust, and my urgency to control things began to dissolve and fade away like little deaths.

And with each little death of these fragmented pieces of my ego "self" came an element of rebirth, eventually allowing more loving and positive thoughts and behaviors to replace them. I began to nourish and heal the hole within, which in the past, I had always tried to fill with something outside myself to ease my inner fears ... including abandonment or the impending loss of a loved one.

These positive changes let me know my true "Self." I went from defining myself by my accomplishments and roles to being more in tune with my heart and what makes me happy and balanced. I will always have an element of my ego mind, but it no longer runs my life or defines my inner sense of 'who I am.'

As I witnessed this cycle of death and rebirth inside myself, I also began to better understand the correlation between meditation and the process of letting go of the physical body. I realized that every time we meditate, we practice the art of dying — a repeated acquaintance with death. It's a constant act of surrendering the intellect of the mind and connecting to the breath, heart, and soul consciousness of the "I am" — potentially in preparation for our own eventual passing.

George Harrison, often described as the "Quiet Beatle," began learning about this connection between meditation and death in his twenties. In the documentary, *Living in the Material World*, his wife, Olivia, talks about George's spiritual relationship with music, his friends, and death. She explains how through his music and lyrics, he cultivated transcendent friendships.

The film is a beautiful portrait of George's life that artfully details highlights of his journey — including his pivotal introduction to Transcendental Meditation® in 1967, which sparked a deep interest and exploration into Eastern philosophy, the practice of meditation, and its eventual relationship to dying.

Over the years, through his religious and spiritual studies, George emphasized the importance of the moment of death and leaving our bodies. Olivia recounts a conversation George had with His Holiness the Dalai Lama about his mindfulness practice. When asked if his practice was working, George replied he wouldn't know until he died.

Based on Olivia's story in the film's last few minutes, she felt his practice had paid off because he could meet that moment without fear, conscious of God, and with an abundance of peace and love within and around him. She describes the moment he left his body as profound — the room was visibly lit up. George passed at a friend's home in Los Angeles with Olivia and his son Dhani by his side.

I share this story with you because it is such a beautiful example of acceptance, surrender, and the intimacy of walking a friend home with love and grace. It's also a profound testament to what meditation can teach us about dropping our bodies and embracing death.

I would never have thought that the simple act of sitting and repeating a mantra would change my life so dramatically, but it has. My daily commitment to meditation has given me an invaluable gift by providing me with a profound tool to navigate stress and embrace life and death with more faith, balance, inner calmness, and a sense of wholeness — a state of being that I would like to be in when my time for transition comes.

Until that happens, I will continue with my moving meditations in nature, as well as my practice of dying through the tradition of Vedic meditation — and live my life more fully and present in every moment to the best of my ability, an experience beyond anything I could have ever imagined for myself.

DADDY: A JOURNEY OF DISCOVERY

Vignette Two

♥

"Today, I will ask myself which direction I am choosing, which part of me I will serve. I will pause to hear the still, small voice within that may encourage me to transcend this animal nature and allow me to give of myself to the world. And no matter how loudly the ego may scream, I will choose at least once today to serve God rather than self." ~ Jeff Kober

A Little History

My dad's story is the longest personal story in this book and my first experience being of service to someone in transition. The year my father was diagnosed with cancer was the year my perception of illness and death changed. I witnessed the truth about the process of dying, something that today I embrace as remarkable.

After my mother died, I went to live with my father and stepmother, Rose. We never discussed that I had just lost my mom or that they would now be responsible for raising a preteen. It was an awkward living situation where I slept in the living room on a pull-out sofa bed for the first year. It was very challenging for all of us. I was essentially living with two strangers.

My father was a kind, quiet man who had been emotionally unavailable for most of my life. I didn't know much about him. One night he got into a car accident on his way home from work, and that's when I learned he had a significant drinking problem. Fortunately, he didn't hurt anyone except himself—lots of cuts and bruises. However, he ended up in jail that night with a DUI.

As part of his punishment, the judge ordered him to attend Alcoholics Anonymous (AA) meetings for 90 days. My father walked through the doors of his first AA meeting and never drank again. I'm happy to say he completed his time here on earth with 29 years of sobriety. That car accident and the resulting sentence were the best things that ever happened to our family.

One of the gifts AA gave my father was a solid spiritual foundation on which he modeled the rest of his life, allowing us to form a supportive relationship. Over time, our bond became so meaningful that I got married on Father's Day. When my daughter Danielle was born, he was among the first to see and hold her. He was very present in both of our lives.

Despite our close relationship, in 1999, Dad chose to keep a potential health issue from me until he could see a doctor. The doctor diagnosed Dad with a respiratory infection and prescribed him antibiotics. Once he knew it wasn't anything serious, he called me to share his scare and the news that he was okay. That was a few days before Thanksgiving, which gave us all a little more to be grateful for that year.

The Labyrinth - Finding Spirituality

Unfortunately, Dad's health didn't improve over the next few months, and he once again kept quiet about how he was feeling. During this period, I had an intuitive vision of a labyrinth in my backyard. When I receive one of these messages, I've learned it's something to pay attention to. I didn't know anything about labyrinths or their purpose, so I decided to do some research. The more I read about these sacred circles' mythology and spiritual and healing abilities, the more I became excited about the idea of creating one.

On February 1, 2000, I began designing and constructing a three-circuit labyrinth with pavers, river rocks, and sand. I didn't realize then what a profound healing tool the entire building process would be for me — on many levels, especially over the next six months.

An Unexpected Diagnosis

A few weeks after I started my project, my father began coughing up blood and experiencing labored breathing and could no longer hide his ill health from us. He went in for a second doctor's opinion in mid-February and learned he had a lung tumor.

Dad had been a smoker from when he was a teenager until he turned 70, which is when my daughter asked him to stop smoking as a gift for her 10th birthday. He loved her so much he would have done anything for her. To my surprise, he obliged and smoked his last cigarette the day before her birthday, five years before the tumor diagnosis.

I believe that when someone develops cancer, it can be a result of different contributing factors influenced by various lifestyle choices:

- Environmental toxins, including pesticides, chemicals, pollution, electromagnetic influences
- Food sources—preservatives, chemicals, synthetic coloring dyes, GMOs
- Smoking

- Genetics
- Emotional stress related to family or work situations.

I think it was the combination of all the above in my father's case. He had carried a lot of stress over the years, not only in raising me, but he was also the primary caregiver for Rose, who had many health issues, and her adult daughter Paula, who had special needs. Rose was older than my father, and somehow, I had always assumed that she would pass first and that my father would have some time to himself to experience a real sense of peace and serenity. As fate would have it, that's not how the story went.

Surgery, Confusion, Denial

The doctor recommended surgery once the test results were in, and my dad agreed. During the operation, they discovered that the cancer cells had already spread into the fluid surrounding his lung. The doctor explained that once cancer reached this advanced stage, it would most likely travel quickly to other parts of his body. He also noted that treatment — not even chemotherapy or radiation — would stop it from spreading,

As I sat there and listened to the doctor's words, I couldn't quite grasp the reality of what I was hearing. I struggled with my feelings and could not conceive of losing my father. What would I do without him? He was my voice of reason, my support team through my divorce, and as a single mother, my best friend, and the wind beneath my wings.

When I got home that night, the only thing that made sense was why I was guided to create a labyrinth. I would need more strength and courage than ever before to accept what the future would bring over the next six months. The sacred circle proved to be that beacon of light, offering me a form of moving meditation and a safe space to express and process my feelings. It was the perfect healing tool for my father and me as we embraced each phase, delivering lessons in patience, trust, faith, letting go, and the importance of meditation.

When Cancer Spreads Quickly

Dad's health appeared to be reasonably good for a few months after the surgery, and we both kept to our daily habits, fitting in a few hours here and there to work in the garden on the labyrinth. Even though I had found acceptance of my dad's illness, a part of me held on to the ray of hope that somehow, I would find a natural solution to kill the cancer cells and save him — a miracle.

Then the phone rang late one night, three months after the diagnosis. It was Dad calling from a phone booth. He was scared and upset but didn't want Rose to know. He said he was feeling strange and having trouble holding onto his keys. I suspected it was a neurological problem related to his cancer and told him not to worry. I then reassured him that I'd come by in the morning to take him to the doctor so they could run some tests.

Unfortunately, I didn't fully understand the severity of the situation until I arrived the next day and saw him sitting on the stairs waiting for me. His appearance and physical abilities had changed dramatically in the few days since I had last seen him. He had gone from being fully functional and self-sufficient to needing someone to help him walk a few steps. He even lost his ability to speak coherently and communicate his basic needs.

The lab where we went for the tests had limited parking access, so I had to drop Dad off at the curb, where an attendant was waiting for him. The test took several hours and confirmed that the cancer cells had spread to his brain. When my father got back in the car that afternoon, I knew in my heart that this, indeed, was the beginning of the end. I remember reaching over, holding his hand in the car, and telling him how much I loved him. I hugged him and assured him I would be there every step of the way to walk him home to a God of his understanding.

At that moment, an array of gifts began to unfold between the two of us. First and foremost, we started a beautiful conversation about our journey together, having gratitude for the experience. We discussed what the latest diagnosis meant and what it might look like moving forward. And finally, we agreed that I would become his death midwife in the preparation and actualization of his journey home.

Our Precious Time Together

In the first few weeks following the new diagnosis, we spent most of our one-on-one time going out for meals near his house. We reminisced about the good times we'd shared and touched on things he wouldn't be around to enjoy with us, like my daughter's milestones. Thankfully, we agreed that he would still be very consciously present in our lives, guiding and watching over us from the other side. We would simply need to learn how to acknowledge that presence and the essence of each other in a new way.

As the weeks went by, we cherished our rare opportunity to speak openly and freely about death and the process of dying, deepening our emotional bond. We made a good father-daughter team.

Dad also continued to ask about the progress of the labyrinth, and we discussed the possibility of it being a portal for our communication after he was gone. Shortly after starting work on it, my daughter and I found a beautiful statue of a Native American goddess with an adolescent girl in her womb and a birdbath pedestal to place her on in the center. We named her Grace. She reminded my daughter and me of our relationship. Together, the two pieces were the perfect centerpiece to harness the energy of the circle. In the beginning stages, I placed her outside the labyrinth, so she could support its creation.

As our father-daughter bond began to dissolve in the physical realm, I found myself connecting to the earth every night through the labyrinth by lighting candles and talking to Grace, who remained watchful over the situation and comforted me.

Prognosis & Treatment

Despite the doctor's prognosis that nothing could cure his cancer, my father decided to undergo radiation treatments. Often when people learn they have a terminal illness, the survival instinct kicks in, and they are willing to try anything — if not for themselves, then for their partner or family members.

While I disagreed with his choice, I did commit to taking him to his treatments. In the first week, something very unexpected happened: my dad's gentle personality turned angry, outspoken, and impatient towards his wife, Rose, and her daughter, Paula. I had never known this aspect of my father and was shocked by his behavior. Thankfully, once he stopped the treatment, his temperament mellowed back out.

One of the downsides of radiation was that my dad deteriorated quickly. If there was a positive to be found in the situation, it was that his cancer had grown in an area of the brain that controlled pain responses — so essentially, he had no pain related to the disease.

When Dad lost all his hair, we both found humor in a baseball cap I gave him with the words "Let's Live" written across the front that served as excellent protection for his now-bald head. His friends loved this silly hat, which would always lighten the mood and spark laughter.

Dad and Rose continued to be somewhat self-sufficient until he started falling frequently, eventually falling in the kitchen one night, severely injuring his hip. When I arrived the next morning and assessed the situation, I immediately called the paramedics and had him transported to the hospital.

At that moment, I realized that my parents could no longer make responsible decisions about their safety. Fortunately, my father had a few weeks' stay in the hospital while he healed. This allowed me to formulate a plan with the doctors about what their next phase would look like.

Finding Humor While Navigating Terminal Illness

Every day was a new experience that brought unknown adventures. At this point, I was the only one who could understand Dad's infantile communication skills, so everyone would anxiously await my arrival to interpret his needs. Some days were hectic, while others were relatively quiet as he straddled between the two worlds of the transition process.

On quiet days, I would read to him from James Van Praagh's book, *Talking to Heaven: A Medium's Message of Life After Death*. He would listen intently to the stories Van Praagh shared about what the spirits had told him over the years from the other side. Dad enjoyed the readings as well as our conversations about them. He often expressed how much he appreciated me and how our talks comforted him about what was to come.

While my life was stressful as a business owner, raising a child, and caring for my dad, the two of us thoroughly embraced the gift of our time together. There were many moments of laughter — essential under challenging circumstances — like the day I got to the hospital and he had lost his dentures. I found them on the hospital floor in the corner of the room behind a privacy drape. When I asked him what had happened, he said he had pushed the button, got in trouble, fell on the floor, and "it hurt." Translation: he had pulled out his catheter tube, which was very painful. He then fell off the bed, further injuring himself and losing his dentures. The night nurse reprimanded him and threatened to tie him to the bed if he didn't behave.

Dad felt so ashamed, but I assured him it was nothing to get worked up over because things like this were bound to happen during this phase. After that episode, whenever I'd leave the hospital, I would turn to him and remind him not to push the button, or he'd get in trouble. He would give me this sheepish look, laugh, and mumble, "I'll be good."

Isolation vs. Community

Sometimes, when people get sick, their loved ones become overly protective of them, and so it was with Rose. She wasn't letting Dad's friends come to visit him. The spiritual fellowship among his AA buddies was so critical and dear to him. Those were the people who knew his deepest, darkest secrets — his authentic self — and with whom he had spent 29 years in recovery. This isolation was a huge loss for my father and his friends.

Eventually, I took a stand and told Rose I thought her actions were unfair. I explained that Dad needed the support of his friends more than ever, and they wanted to be part of the process. At first, Rose resisted, but eventually, she came around and opened the door to those closest to him.

Waiting for Ida

As things progressed, I called my father's only living sister Ida to let her know the state of his health. Ida was in her 80s but still spry and working five days a week. I asked her if she wanted to come say goodbye to Dad, and she agreed.

When I asked if he wanted to see Ida, his eyes lit up. I explained she couldn't come for another two weeks and asked if he would still be with us. He looked up at the ceiling and thought about it for a long time before he finally smiled and said, "Tell her we have a date."

When I arrived the following morning, Dad appeared to be slipping away into an unfamiliar kind of sleep. His movements were strange, and he made odd mumbling sounds. Periodically he would open his eyes, and when I asked him where he was, he told me he was at "The Man's Party." (He used to refer to his Higher Power as "The Man.") Dad also kept talking about the birds. Based on his behavior, I thought he would surely die that day. I even had a friend bring my daughter to the hospital.

My daughter and I sat with Dad holding his hand for hours and talking. Occasionally he would wake up and answer us, then return to communing with the spirit world. Each time it happened, we would both giggle with amazement at bearing witness to this odd yet intriguing experience. We decided he was at God's party, and the birds were angels. Eventually, we left him at the party and went home to rest. The nurse assured me he would call if there were any changes during the night.

I returned to the hospital early the following day, only to find Dad sitting up and feeding himself.

"What are you doing?" I asked.

"I'm eating breakfast; why?" Dad replied.

When I told him that I thought he was going to leave us yesterday, he said, "Oh no, it takes some getting used to. You have to come and go a lot before you finally go."

Dad continued to explain that the "propralees" (some type of being he saw or connected with on the other side) assisted him in feeling comfortable with the process. It pleased him that there was guidance every step of the way and that I was interested in learning all about it.

Dad's Homecoming & Preparing for Transition

The following day, after speaking with his doctor, we all agreed it was time to take him home and bring in a nurse and hospice. This action would also remedy the situation of Rose being alone and vulnerable. Dad was happy to be headed home, where he would be more comfortable in his last days.

As his condition continued deteriorating, I wasn't sure he would make it until his sister arrived. But over the next week, every night before I left, I told Dad how many more days there were until Ida would arrive. And then I'd ask if he'd be there when I returned in the morning. Every night he would briefly pause, move into thought by looking upward, and then smile and shake his head yes.

Dad slept most of the time in those final weeks. Many of his close friends began visiting him regularly to express gratitude for their relationships. Even though he was weak and tired, he looked forward to the visits and updates on the happenings in the AA rooms. The opportunity to connect with his friends was a gift for them all.

We continued our open discussion about the process, confirming that once his physical body was gone, we would still find ways to communicate. These conversations made Dad feel more comfortable about dying, and he was grateful I took the time to explain things to him in the best way I could with my limited knowledge.

Moving From Fear & Denial into Acceptance Without Regrets

Once Dad was home, he also started experiencing visitations from some of his friends and family members who had passed years before him, so I knew his time here was nearing completion. The only thing he was waiting for was his sister's arrival.

Despite Dad's progression, Rose was still living in a complete state of fear and denial that he would soon be gone. When people came to visit, she didn't want anyone to discuss that he was dying, especially not in front of him. I tried to explain to her the importance of being able to talk about what was happening so that he would feel supported and safe, but she couldn't grasp that concept.

As we moved into the final days, I expressed my feelings to Rose about the importance of having that last honest conversation with her husband before he was gone. I didn't want her to have any regrets. The hospice team and social workers all reiterated my thoughts, and then we left her alone to process the idea.

The next morning, when I arrived Rose was sitting in the kitchen crying. My father had initiated a conversation with her but she didn't want to discuss it. Dad was weak and resting, but the caregiver told me he had overheard my father tell Rose she shouldn't wait too long before joining him after he was gone.

I held Rose as she wept and affirmed that I was happy they could share that intimacy and completion. It was so painful and bittersweet, but I knew any denial or question Rose might have had concerning Dad's status was now gone.

Tools for Emotional Self-care

Some of the tools that helped me stay present and connected during this incredibly stressful time (other than the labyrinth) were journaling about our experiences together and periodically pulling a card from one of my inspirational card decks. I frequently used them to set the day's tone. Not everyone feels comfortable using these tools, but I have always resonated with them for their potential insights and guidance.

A week after Dad came home, I sat down to meditate and felt drawn to pull seven cards. I left them all face down, and each morning, I would turn over the next top card on the pile and read its daily message. The reading was always very synchronistic with the day ahead, fueling me to stay strong and balanced.

Ida's Arrival & Goodbye

Finally, the day came for Ida to arrive. I picked her up at the airport and did my best to prepare her to see her brother. For those of us who saw my father daily, the physical changes were gradual.

However, I knew it might be very traumatic for someone who hadn't seen him in years. And it was.

My aunt's generation didn't readily talk about or acknowledge feelings and emotions, so I knew saying goodbye to her dear "Danny Boy" wouldn't be easy.

Ida spent two days with Dad, where he remained slumbering most of the time, only opening his eyes briefly now and then to reconnect with her.

When it came time for the final goodbye, Ida kept repeating, "So long, Danny Boy. I love you, and I'll see you soon."

I could see by the look on Dad's face that he thought she meant she'd be back the next day, but I knew he was exhausted and wasn't interested in sticking around much longer.

After she left the room, I held his hand and clarified that Ida had difficulty saying goodbye and that he would not be seeing her again in his lifetime. Dad's last wish had been fulfilled, and he told me he understood.

When I arrived the following morning, Dad was panting and said he was frightened. His caregiver also pointed out that his lower extremities had turned blue up to his knees as his circulatory system began to shut down (similar to a newborn waiting for their circulatory system to integrate after cutting the umbilical cord).

As I sat there comforting him, I realized leaving this world was much like coming into the world. It requires a type of laboring as you try to let go of your body, similar to the birthing process, separating from your mother and emerging from her womb. This somatic occurrence affirmed the interconnectedness of the birthing and dying process.

Dad whispered, "I don't like this part," and I told him I would get him something to make the process easier. He looked at me with relief, laughed, and said, "Please hurry."

My daughter and her father arrived a few minutes later to say their final goodbyes. Once they left, I gave Dad the medication that hospice sent over and told him again how much I loved and appreciated him being my father and what an honor it was to have been his daughter.

He looked into my eyes and whispered one last faint, "I love you too. We made a good team."

A few minutes later, he relaxed into a deep, peaceful sleep. As I walked away that night, I knew our journey together was complete. I cried all the way home, not so much in sadness but for the gift of our relationship.

Letting Go

When I got home, I couldn't sleep in anticipation of the call telling me he was gone, so I began journaling. Around 4:00 a.m., I realized I still had one card left in my stack. When I turned it over, this is what it said:

"Letting Go — In this image of lotus leaves in the early morning, we can see in the rippling of the water that one drop has just fallen. It is a precious moment and one that is full of poignancy. In surrendering to gravity and slipping off the

leaf, the drop loses its previous identity and joins the vastness of the water below."[2]

We can imagine that it must have trembled before it fell, just on the edge between the known and the unknowable. To choose this card is a recognition that something is finished, something is completing. Whatever it is — a job, a relationship, a home you have loved, anything that might have helped you to define who you are — it is time to let go of it, allowing any sadness, but not trying to hold on.

Something greater is awaiting you. New dimensions are there to be discovered. You are past the point of no return now, and gravity is doing its work. Go with it — it represents liberation."

As I reflected on these words, I realized I had also come to the last page of my journal and knew at that moment, deep in my soul, that my father had been released from his body. A phone call shortly thereafter confirmed my feeling. His leaving was gentle and peaceful, just like his personality.

---

[2] Osho Zen Tarot ~ The Transcendental Game of Zen. Published 1994 St. Martin's Press. Page 112/Commentary text "Letting Go" reprinted with permission from OSHO International.

The Labyrinth, Opening the Portal

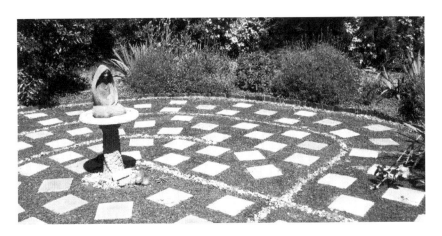

On the day of his passing, I asked my daughter and a few friends to help me lift Grace onto her pedestal in the middle of the labyrinth. We lit a candle and said a prayer for my father as we opened the portal for the communication that he and I often spoke about in his last six months. While the labyrinth was still in its beginning stages at the time, it now had a solid center from which to work and hold the space for my father's energy.

CHAPTER 3

MAKING FRIENDS WITH DEATH

To make friends with death, or any fear, we must first be willing to acknowledge it and then be willing to talk about it. In this section, we'll explore the fear of death and become more comfortable with the subject by opening the doors to honest conversations. When we can be authentic about our feelings and connect with our loved ones about them, there is an opportunity to experience a rare form of intimacy and connection.

The Vibrational Frequency of Emotions - Love & Fear

All emotions and thoughts carry different vibrational frequencies that either support a state of pleasure or create suffering. The scientific support for "vibrational energy" has been well documented and is available through online searches of "the vibrational frequency of thoughts and emotions."

The two most prominent emotions in life are love and fear. Love is the divine force of moving energy that flows in and out of our hearts, uniting consciousness and the material world. It is a catalyst for faith, flow, and connection and energetically holds a high frequency of light that produces a state of wholeness within.

Fear, on the other hand, has two aspects — the first is a primal intuitive alarm system that signals us of impending danger and triggers our nervous system into '"fight, flight, freeze, fawn"' mode to protect us. This aspect of fear is known as a "right action" response and is essential for our safety — when we are, in fact, in danger.

The flip side to this innate warning system occurs when people become preoccupied or obsessed with continuous fear-based thoughts, often from some form of media, others' fears, or unidentified or unprocessed feelings. This negative side of fear vibrates at a lower frequency and can cause undue psychological, physical, social, and/or emotional stress and suffering.

Inherently, we are born with love, the higher vibration, and maintain this lightness of spirit until life events and our ego-mind begin to *manufacture* fear. These thought processes are often a modeled behavior, sometimes passed down generationally, setting us up for an unhealthy pattern of anxiety around certain subjects — death being one of them.

As an only child in a single (working) parent household, I spent a lot of time alone or at friends' homes after school. I remember having a lot of anxious feelings — sensations in my body and unwanted thoughts in my mind — that I didn't understand. Sometimes, I felt something was wrong with me, but I didn't know who to talk to about it. When I think back, I don't remember ever hearing any conversations about feelings between adults and children (of any age) with friends or family members.

The Conversation

That type of avoidance and silence around feelings is common for people of my generation. Like my parents, many adults were never taught how to acknowledge or talk about their feelings, nor were they given tools to process them. Consequently, many adults today still have trouble expressing their thoughts and fears and don't know how to model a healthy conversation about them with their families.

A few years ago, I saw an inspiring movie, *It's A Beautiful Day in the Neighborhood*, based on a true story about Fred Rogers (the creator of the children's show *Mr. Rogers' Neighborhood*) and his relationship with journalist Tom Junod. The film offered viewers a message of kindness, love, and forgiveness and reminded me of Rogers' unique role as a teacher to both adults and children.

Mr. Rogers' Neighborhood taught people how to connect with their feelings and process them using mindful conversations between human beings (in real-life situations) and puppets in a world of make-believe. One day when he found his goldfish dead during the show, Rogers used the opportunity to talk about how sad he was that his friend had died. This was the first time anyone had publicly spoken directly to children about death and the feelings associated with it.

Rogers explained how having these uncomfortable feelings was normal and not something to be ignored or dismissed. He encouraged the kids to talk about them — fear, anger, sadness, disappointment, etc. — so their thoughts would become more manageable. He went on to reminisce about losing his childhood dog, Mitzy, and assured the kids that these feelings wouldn't last forever.

Having these types of healthy conversations with anyone helps us process our feelings and helps others understand what we are going through so they can better support us as well. I believe Rogers' example of these social and emotional practices is an essential teaching tool for all ages, especially concerning death.

"When we can talk about our feelings, they become less overwhelming, less upsetting, and less scary. The people we trust with that important talk can help us know that we're not alone." ~ Fred Rogers[3]

When people get caught in the lower frequency of their fear of death, a sense of disconnection, separateness, or fragmentation of the spirit often arises, depriving them of the opportunity to connect with the people they love. I know this fear and deprivation firsthand because of the silence in my family when my mother was dying of cancer. Consequently, she and I missed out on a lot of important mother-daughter conversations.

There were so many things I would have liked to know about her life experiences, our heritage, or a chance to fill in the gaps of my childhood memories before she died, all of which were lost. There was no opportunity to talk about our feelings to help either of us process them or share moments of intimacy with each other. My mother and I took that journey separately, leaving me with tremendous unprocessed grief and a huge void in my heart.

The Origin: Fear of Death

Let's take a closer look at the act of dying. There are only a few ways death comes upon us: old age, a random accident, an unexpected health-related event, a violent incident, suicide, or a terminal illness. When we die of old age, it is more accepted, expected, and sometimes welcomed. An elderly person has presumably lived a full life, and their body is ready for retirement. Conversely, when someone is taken away from us unexpectedly,

---

[3] Fred Rogers, quote reprinted with permission from Fred Rogers Productions, Licensing Dept.

which can happen at any age, it feels like we are biologically cheated out of time.

Death is a mystery because it is a dance with the unknown. We often develop a fear of dying at our first conscious concept of what the word means, depending on its presentation and by whom we learned about it.

The fear of death is often established in childhood through the family unit, culture, or religion. It can also result from witnessing a traumatic event or someone else's visceral reaction to the situation or death. A visual and/or audio memory of this nature can be permanently imprinted in your mind, especially if your feelings about the experience are not properly identified, addressed, and processed.

Recognizing uncomfortable feelings about death, including loss, sadness, anxiety, anger, and abandonment, is the first step in addressing them. One of the most common fears is not knowing where we go when we die. People are scared of the unknown, the vulnerability, or the impermanence of their mortality.

When considering another person's death, the overwhelming factor is often the anticipation of the emptiness we'll feel when that person is gone or the potential for witnessing a loved one's physical/emotional pain as they go through their process. Other times, it's the discomfort of considering our own death — an early grieving of the things we will miss out on when we are gone, the thought of experiencing our own physical/emotional pain, or the guilt of leaving someone whom we have cared for and believe still needs us. There are many different reasons why people fear death.

When my daughter was young, one of my girlfriends who had twin daughters introduced the three of them (and me) to death as a cycle of life through the book *Charlotte's Web*. The girls were all under two, and it proved to be a healthy way of planting seeds for future discussions throughout their childhood. All three of these girls have grown into strong, independent women who have a sense of peace about dying and death. Yes, they still have fears, but they are reasonable and balanced concerns based on their childhood experiences. (See "Pam's Gift from the Universe")

Identifying and Processing Fear: Exercises & Resources

I encourage you to take the time to get clear about your feelings about death. If you explore where your fears come from by asking yourself the following questions, you can begin to better understand these feelings. Once you've established the answers, you will feel more relaxed about opening up a dialog with others, especially your kids, using similar questions to explore their feelings — tailored to their age readiness (young, midlife, or even those preparing for transition).

- What are my beliefs about death?
- Are they based on my religion or spiritual practices?
- When and where did I learn about death? What was the circumstance of that memory?
- What is it that I am so afraid of? Can I put my fear into words?
- Where do we go when we die?
- Have I accepted that death is inevitable?
- What steps and actions can I take to change my thoughts about death?

Asking these questions is a constructive way of searching for your truth. When you begin to reflect on these questions, you will probably come up with more questions of your own. Take time to explore your feelings around them. After losing my mother at such a young age, I did a lot of soul-searching to heal in this area. Some of the actions that helped me cultivate a healthier relationship with my fears about death included the following three things, plus some of the following resources:

- Talking openly about death with others and asking questions like, "What do you want to know about death?"
- Being of service to those in transition with an open mind and heart — facing the inevitable with forgiveness, compassion, and courage
- Implementing a meditation practice that allows me to better understand the process of my own body and life cycle

Again, if the subject of death is left in the shadows, it will continue to be a dark, scary thing. But if you bring death into the room, infuse it with some light, and acknowledge its inevitability, you may find that this fear begins to dissolve. This is what I call making friends with death.

Let's break this generational fear of death together and start the conversation.

Tools for Addressing Fear

It is always best to do your own research and check with a qualified healthcare provider before starting any new modality or protocol. The following tools have proven to be successful for many dealing with different emotional situations, including fears around death and feeling anxious, as well as for those in transition or those caring for someone in their last phase of life:

Emotional Freedom Technique — EFT

Emotional Freedom Technique or EFT is a tapping technique based on the combined principles of ancient Chinese acupressure and modern psychology. It creates a form of psychological acupressure. It works by tapping on a series of Chinese acupressure points called "meridians" on the body in a specific sequence while thinking about the negative thoughts that bother you. Research shows that tapping on these points as you verbally express your feelings or think about them can calm the amygdala in the brain to regulate the nervous system and immediately reduce stress and anxiety. The technique can be used anywhere, anytime, with any age group to help relieve emotional distress.

You can use EFT to manage a wide range of everyday emotions — anger, resentment, fear, sadness, anxiety, stress, trauma, PTSD, and pre-test jitters, among others. While I had known about EFT for years through the studies and writings of medical researcher Dawson Church, I didn't start using the technique in my personal or professional life until 2012. That day came when I met Nick Ortner at a Hay House Conference and witnessed firsthand, EFT's powerful healing abilities.

Ortner founded The Tapping Solution and produces an annual free online event called the Tapping World Summit, which teaches people how to use EFT daily. In 2013, he also created The Tapping Solution Foundation in response to his local community's needs after the Sandy Hook Elementary School shooting to help them emotionally heal from this horrific trauma. Their organization provides many community services to all types of groups — schools, vets, hospitals, and so on.

I use EFT every day and have seen the miracles it produces for myself, as well as with my clients.

Bach Flower Essence Remedies

Flower Essence remedies are also a wonderful tool to help people of all ages deal with emotional disharmony — minor or major upset. They are made from flower buds, blossoms, and clippings of wild bushes, plants, and trees. The sun's light infuses the flora in spring water, creating an energetic imprint of their healing essence. The flower remedies have no taste or smell, are non-toxic, and have no side effects.

In the 1930s, Dr. Edward Bach, an English scientist, bacteriologist, and practicing physician, discovered that he could shift his emotional state from discomfort to balance just by being around certain plants. He spent the following six years learning about the benefits of different plants and studying their effects on his patients' moods.

Dr. Bach found that a person's physical symptoms would heal by treating the body as a whole — mind, body, and spirit. As a result of his work, he developed the 38 Bach Flower remedies. The most famous essence used worldwide today is Rescue Remedy, a combination of five different Bach flower essences successfully used on humans (and animals) of all ages — with no side effects — to help relieve emotional suffering.

For more information about EFT and Bach Flower Essence remedies, please see the Resource section.

Essential Oils & Aromatherapy for Fears

A word of caution: It is important to use essential oils properly. Even though they are made from natural extracts, certain oils can irritate or injure eyes, mucous membranes, cause photosensitivity, and should not be worn or left on the skin in direct sunlight; others may cause skin irritation if applied directly to the skin. Always read the package or consult a qualified practitioner before use, especially if you have underlying medical conditions or are pregnant. The author and publisher disclaim all responsibility for any effects that may occur due to the mention or context in this book.

Essential oils are made from compounds extracted from the bark, flowers, leaves, stems, roots, and other parts of plants that are put through one of several various distillation processes — what remains is an essential oil.

Aromatherapy is a holistic healing treatment using essential oil(s) through several different methods: applied to the skin directly in droplets, added to an oil carrier for massage, diffused into the air, placed in a bath, and so on. Their healing energy and aromatic scents can be very strong and should be used with care, as some people may be sensitive to them or find them too overpowering.

Different oils provide different benefits for people on both an emotional (i.e., fears, anxiety, depression) and physical level (i.e., antibacterial, antiviral, fevers, earaches) The aromatic scent of essential oils impacts the brain's limbic system, which controls emotions, certain physiological functions (i.e., heart rate, breathing), smell, and memory.

The most common essential oils used to calm stress, anxiety, and fears include:

Chamomile: Provides a calming effect on the mind and body and soothes anxious feelings.

FrankIncense: Relieves anxiety and fear to help us get grounded, find clarity, and connect with our intuition.

Geranium: Helps open our hearts and can assist in restoring our faith and managing overwhelming emotions; also helpful for anxiety and depression.

Juniper: Gives us the courage to take appropriate actions to address our fears and anxiety.

Lavender: Alleviates stress, fear, sadness, and emotional trauma; it can bring clarity to a situation and assist with honest and open communication.

Sweet Orange: reduces worry, stress, fear, anxiety, and depression

ROSE: MY STEPMOTHER

Vignette Three

♥

To love, especially at those times when we seem least capable of it, is to build a muscle that will serve us the rest of our life."
~ *Jeff Kober*

Finding Forgiveness & Healing Resentments Through Acts of Service

My relationship with my stepmother, Rose (and her daughter, Paula), was complicated, and her care was the most difficult for me. There were many times I wanted to run away and hide, but I promised my father I would take care of her and Paula, and I knew in my heart it was the right thing to do.

Their stories describe some of the emotions and feelings I felt on my journey of self-discovery and healing through this challenging act of service. I created a safe space for their vulnerability and cared for their needs, even when they couldn't fully appreciate my actions or may not have been able to do the same if our roles were reversed. Sometimes, their requests were for something major, while other times, they just wanted to be seen, heard, and supported.

There was a lot of laughter, sadness, anger, grief, reflection, and then surrender, acceptance, and letting go. What I realized through this process was that none of us had grown up in a positive nurturing environment or received healthy forms of affection or emotional support from our parents — something I believe I was able to give each of them a glimpse of — and experience myself — in their final days.

To my surprise, I learned how to listen to their needs and concerns differently, with a softer heart, eventually loving and appreciating these two women through the bitterness and resentment of our past. (Also, see Paula's story.)

These experiences showed me it's never too late to learn how to love someone and that love itself is a wonderful tool for healing and fostering forgiveness — for all parties involved, even if we don't realize it until they are gone.

> *"You forgive to free yourself. It's not important who is right or wrong."* ~ Brené Brown [4]

Rose wasn't a wicked stepmother, but she wrestled with tremendous jealousy, pain, and resentment from her childhood. Her parents died when she was 12, and she ended up living with her sister and brother-in-law, a man who liked to drink. Without a nurturing parental role model, Rose had no concept of how to show or express familial love, which, unfortunately, was reflected in our lifelong turbulent relationship with each other.

Despite all the dysfunction and challenges between us, Rose was a gift to my father and me. She was instrumental in creating a strong, ethical balance in our family, which is something for which I will always be grateful.

---

[4] Brown, B. (2017). Rising Strong: How the Ability to Reset Transforms the Way We Live, Love, Parent, and Lead. Random House. Quote reprinted in compliance with BrenéBrown.com permission guidelines.

When I first met Rose, she was a prominent hairdresser at the Beverly Wilshire Hotel, a landmark featured in the movie *Pretty Woman*. By the time I moved in with her and my father, she had already had two heart attacks and could no longer work. This never seemed to slow her down. She was always on top of things, especially keeping a watchful eye on me — a young teen. My father used to refer to her as the "detective."

Rose was plagued with many illnesses and mishaps through the years — lung cancer, more heart attacks, colon cancer, and broken bones. We eventually dubbed her the "Energizer Bunny." No matter what physical challenge appeared, she just kept right on going.

My father was the one with a strong constitution, but as you already know, he ended up dying before Rose, and I inherited the job of being responsible for her.

One of Dad's words of wisdom to me was that Rose and I would work out our differences. I had my doubts, but as usual, he was right — albeit not without some begrudging final challenges.

Three weeks after Dad died, Rose, then 83, suffered what the doctors labeled another mild heart attack, and she ended up in the hospital. Thankfully, this gave me a little time to grieve the loss of my father and formulate a plan for her care.

During her hospital stay, the doctors discovered that her lung cancer had returned. They told us there was nothing they could do for her, and we all decided the best course of action was to send her home to hospice. That plan would provide her with a safe environment of continuous care in the comfort of her own home without any dramatic lifestyle changes.

My only experience with hospice was with my father's care in his final two weeks, which was incredibly positive. He was also a kind, passive, and accepting man who was an easy patient and at ease with dying, whereas Rose was not — quite the opposite. Knowing her temperament and how she needed to control things, I wasn't sure how long she might live. Moreover, with her history, as well as our dysfunctional relationship, I knew it wasn't going to be easy.

The main difference between my father's and Rose's situation was that I knew what he was waiting for to feel complete (his sister's visit), and I had no idea what it would take for her to feel that sense of completion. Rose's situation seemed different. There wasn't any unfinished business — no relatives to say goodbye to or tasks to complete. After much reflection, the only thing I could think of was how codependent Rose was with her special needs daughter, Paula.

Rose was fearful that no one would have the emotional patience or knowledge to properly care for Paula. Consequently, her resistance to letting go appeared to be more about trust — not just in general, but specifically in me. My intuition told me Rose was waiting for her faith and trust in me to arrive, and I knew that could take some time.

A Process of Separation

Once Rose was home from the hospital, my daily morning responsibilities entailed ensuring all her needs were met and that she was comfortable. Paula and the caregiver would take over in the afternoon when I'd go home to catch up on work and care for my daughter.

My experience of being of service to Rose was much more complicated than it had been with my father. As time passed and her body weakened, her usual nasty behavior escalated into unacceptable abuse. Eventually, I could no longer give of myself without feeling stressed and resentful, and I knew something would have to change for me to continue helping her.

I called Harold, the hospice social worker, and asked for help. He explained that Rose's behavior was quite normal as she began her process of separation from both me and especially her daughter. Thankfully, Harold was willing to step in and have an appropriate conversation with Rose about her feelings and behavior. His sage words regarding the process of dying helped her feel a little safer and less fearful and soothed some of my resentment. He was an angel of patience and instrumental in helping us resolve the issue and find some semblance of peace in our relationship. It was after that conversation that Rose began to soften and trust me.

Surrender & Letting Go

Through the years, I've also observed that people who are comfortable with the process of dying relish having their loved ones close during the final days and weeks, whereas those who fear the mystery of death or don't have a spiritual base need their space. Rose was the latter.

Once Rose became more comfortable with embracing death, there was a distinct surrender to her process of letting go. She began to get frequent visits from spirit beings, many of whom were strangers that she described only by gender. When my father started visiting her regularly, I knew it wouldn't be long before they would be reunited.

I remember my father talking about the process of transition as something that takes some getting used to — a type of integration process where the person comes and goes a lot before they make that final crossing.

No Goodbye for Paula

Even though Paula didn't always intellectually understand things, she was very intuitive and lived in the present moment. Her main concerns were about how she would navigate her day versus what might be happening in the future. She lived in a world of repetitive behavior — always asking the same questions over and over every day, which usually precipitated a fight between Rose and her.

Rose and my father kept many things from Paula because she was easily upset and confused. I decided that after a lifetime of being sheltered from reality, it was time to tell Paula the truth about her mom — that she wasn't going to get better this time and that she was preparing to die.

Her response was surprising. She said, "I know," and that was the end of it. She never talked about it with Rose and continued her daily routine of showing up and sitting with her dying mother.

Rose never brought it up. Upon reflection, I think Rose's silence may have been because she thought by dying, she was letting Paula down, failing, or even abandoning her in some way. Rose's fear often seemed to overshadow her love, a love I knew she had deep in her heart under that rough exterior.

Honoring Rose & Forgiveness — A Cherished Moment

Rose's final day came on a brisk winter evening in January. I arrived mid-morning to a peaceful setting in the apartment. She was resting with a smile on her face, and her caregiver, Norma, said she had been talking to my father most of the night. She hadn't eaten in a few days and spent most of her time sleeping. I knew she would leave us soon.

Norma had just given Rose a sponge bath, dressed her in her favorite pink nightgown, and put fresh sheets on the bed. As I walked by the room, I heard Rose say, "This feels good, but I'm cold."

Harold arrived mid-afternoon, along with another gentleman who was training. The three of us sat in Rose's room, observing and discussing how beautiful she looked at that moment. She must have heard us because she briefly opened her eyes, stared at an empty chair in the corner, and asked, "What are all of you handsome men doing here?" We laughed in acknowledgment, and I told her they were there to welcome her home. She smiled.

What happened next was one of my most cherished memories the two of us would share. Rose turned her head and looked at me with a depth in her eyes that emanated pure divine love. It was a connection and exchange of energy I had never encountered in our 40-year relationship. All the past resentments of our challenging stepmother-daughter experience seemed to disappear as I looked into her eyes and softly said, "I love you."

As her eyes connected with mine for our last defining moment in this lifetime, the words flowed back to me with ease in a whisper, "I love you, too."

Rose transitioned a few hours later in the peace of her own home. Then and now, I am so grateful for Rose and all the lessons our relationship taught me.

CHAPTER 4

UNDERSTANDING THE CYCLE OF LIFE:
BIRTH, LIFE, DEATH

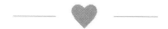

As a mother and student of life, I've spent the last forty years learning how to make conscious decisions that align with the laws of nature and my heart. Living this type of intentional lifestyle requires education and an awareness of how our choices affect our families, others, and the planet.

This approach to decision-making helps us find our truth rather than continuing to follow traditional family patterns or surrendering to peer pressure. These choices will inevitably impact all areas of our lives, including the birthing process and how we prepare for death.

In this chapter, I will focus on the consciousness aspect of birth, life, and death and share my thoughts about where we come from, where we go when we die, and how a person's life plan and views about life and death are shaped.

My opinions are based on my own spiritual practices, in-depth research, and personal experiences from greeting newborns and assisting those in transition as they cross over at the end of their lives. So please take what you can relate to and leave the rest.

Conception: Where Do We Come From?

To better understand the process of death, we must first identify our own thoughts about where we come from and where we might go when we die. We never talked about things like this when I was growing up, so it took a lot of soul-searching to come to my conclusions.

It's hard to say when life begins or ends because there are always going to be varied thoughts about these two complex questions. There are some people whose ideas will be influenced by their own family's beliefs, while others will seek and form their truth — as I did.

I believe a soul's consciousness is not something that is tangible but rather eternal energy that exists before birth and continues after death. I am not a scientist, so the best way I can describe what I believe happens at the moment of conception and moment of death is connected to the seen and unseen worlds — a relationship between matter, energy, and the interconnectedness of all things in all dimensions.

The interconnectedness of the *Material World* & *Quantum Field* - together creating a whole

Matter: *physical body*	Energy: *the soul*
seen	unseen
material form	infinite space
managed time	no time
science	unproven
intellect	intuition/spiritual
visible	invisible/indivisible
existence	non-existence

Science itself is based on the material world (matter), and the quantum field of the universe is dimensional — an infinite expanse of energy and frequencies. When a soul's consciousness comes into the world, it merges with this matter at conception and enters the physical body creating form. This soul-body convergence will remain as one throughout its life cycle until the body dies and the soul is once again released from its physical form back into the infinite energetic field of the universe as a continuum of consciousness.

A soul's ultimate purpose is to transform and grow spiritually by mastering different karmic lessons. Karma is the spiritual balance of cause and effect and plays an intrinsic part in the equation of reincarnation. For those who believe in this concept, each cycle of birth and death is considered an incarnation. Reincarnation is the repetition of this cycle where a soul journeys into and out of a new body (or form), throughout multiple lifetimes — if indeed you do return to form. Reincarnation's meaning differs between ideologies.

A person's karma is based on a law of reciprocity — an exchange of the energy of giving and receiving. What you put out will always come back to you, and your actions in this and previous lives will inevitably play a part in the fate of your future incarnations.

Perhaps you have heard someone describing another person as having negative or positive karma. People with good karma presumably have worked through some of their more difficult life lessons and are living according to their heart's purpose, as opposed to those who are here in this lifetime to sort out their old patterns of struggle. Neither is bad nor good — it is just their lesson this time around.

Another element of a soul's journey is found within the framework of a predetermined karmic plan and contract with the Divine (i.e.,

God, Spirit, Jesus, the Lord, Buddha, Nature, or whatever word you prefer), which dictates our life path. In addition to that contract, we also have karmic agreements with every person we meet in each lifetime — a family member, friend, spouse, child, or even a stranger. Each one plays a role in helping you fulfill your destiny throughout your evolution — intertwining all of these life cycles.

Have you ever wondered why someone seems familiar to you when you have never met them? Or have you ever had a feeling that you've been in a particular situation before, having that very conversation with the same person? The French call this 'déjà vu', or "already seen." While science has no answer to where this experience comes from, I believe this to be a memory of a past life, a soul's connection.

Once your soul has achieved its goal and completed what it came here to do, it is then released from the physical body back to Spirit at the moment of death. A soul never dies ... it simply represents a state of impermanence.

"The way you live life today will inevitably influence the way you will choose to prepare for death." ~ Kathy Arnos

Birth & Welcoming A Spirit

The decision to have a baby comes with a lot of responsibility. If a soul truly begins its cycle of life at conception, it makes sense that how we are conceived and brought into this world is important. Once we have this knowledge, it is up to us to choose whether we will do it with conscious intention or not. Each family makes their decision based on what is right for them. Either way, babies will continue to be born, live, and survive (and hopefully thrive).

Research today suggests that the in-utero experience and how a baby presents itself to the world (i.e., head first, breach, "sunny side up," C-section, natural, induced) can influence the development of one's personality, identity, physical and emotional behaviors, and life patterns.

The Secret Life of the Unborn Child: How You Can Prepare Your Baby for a Happy, Healthy Life by Dr. Thomas Verny explains how a fetus can see, hear, experience, taste, and even learn in utero. The psychological aspects of their pre- and perinatal experiences will range within individual family dynamics from traumatic to serene based on different events and a mother's interactions with others during pregnancy — i.e., dancing, swimming, walking, abusive situations, stressful encounters, or soothing experiences — impacting the developing fetus.

The Birth

The creation and birth of a newborn is a true miracle. Babies are usually born curious, responsive, and alert. One of our first responsibilities is to help them feel safe and affirm their sense of belonging as they integrate into their new environment.

Being present at this extraordinary occurrence of birth is something you'll never forget (as is being present at someone's death.) It can be messy, sometimes complicated and overwhelming, yet one of the most incredible wonders of life.

Regardless of the circumstances surrounding the birth, that newborn arrives helpless and dependent on someone else to care for all of its needs, requiring unconditional love, nurturing, and security. Some receive this type of care — and others do not.

This nurturing response establishes fundamental personality traits formed around healthy or unhealthy attachment patterns developed in childhood. Attachment is a word used by psychologists to describe the relationship between children and their caregivers. If a child's needs are not adequately met or *they feel like they weren't met*, this may influence their overall relationships as they age.

This act of love and care usually comes full circle when we are in the last phase of life, once again requiring someone else to meet our needs.

The Welcoming

Consciously welcoming a new soul to earth is another important element. I have had the honor of being present at dozens of births, and my favorite part is welcoming this newborn to our physical plane. I do this with a simple, intentional greeting: "Welcome to this world." There is nothing more satisfying than getting a smile in response.

I then offer them a blessing (either aloud or silently) and tell them how happy we are that they have arrived, how lucky they are to have chosen their parents, and how fortunate their parents are to have received them. I believe this ritual is comforting and offers a newborn a sense of balance in that transitional moment from the womb to the external world.

I feel as strongly about this welcoming message as I do, about delivering a similar loving message of completion at the end of life. I have found this supportive exchange of words to be equally soothing to those in transition. Examples of this are expressed throughout this book.

The following short story exemplifies the importance of this type of communication at birth. Years ago, my boyfriend's good friend and his wife had a baby boy, and while I don't know all of the details about his in-utero experience or birth, he was born with leukemia. The parents were fear-stricken, and doctors weren't very hopeful about his life expectancy. Knowing the family's religious beliefs, the doctor suggested they have the baby christened as soon as possible. My boyfriend was asked to be his godfather, and I was invited to the ceremony as well.

When we arrived at the church, the infant sat quietly in his car seat on a side table. Although several adults, including me, were trying to engage with him, he didn't make eye contact with any of us. I offered to watch him while the others took care of some last-minute details before the ceremony.

I sat with this beautiful little soul and welcomed him to the world, assuring him that he was very much loved and wanted. I spoke about why he might have come in with this illness and his purpose here, adding that the choice to stay or leave was entirely up to him.

When I finished, he looked up at me and gave me a big smile. At that moment, his mother rejoined us, saying he rarely, if ever, had made eye contact with others and expressed what a joy it was to see him smile. Ultimately, her little boy chose to stay, and within the first year, he was healthy and thriving.

While we'll never know whether that conversation played a part in his recovery, there was nothing to lose by offering him my thoughts and spending a little time with him. I do, however, believe that he and I fulfilled some type of contract with each other that day.

To learn more about pre- and perinatal psychology, see Resources.

Meeting Our True Self

The middle phase of life predominantly revolves around our personalities, identity, and getting to know our deeper selves. As mentioned in the previous section, there are many contributing factors to this development of self.

Even our parents' generational upbringing plays a part based on their childhood experiences and home environment — addiction and abuse versus calm and nurturing. They, in turn, unconsciously pass these traits down to us. While our parents' actions aren't always the reason that we possess positive or negative characteristics, they do strongly influence our personalities.

Our identities, on the other hand, develop more through our life experiences, vocations, and accomplishments. They can also be influenced by our roles within the family, societal dynamics, spiritual or religious practices, and relationships, including with ourselves.

The 20s, 30s, and 40s are the formative years of adulthood when people are busy creating a foundation, raising families, and learning how to navigate life with a sense of efficiency. Whether we simply survive or thrive during this period will depend on our relationships with others, ourselves, and the world around us.

To figure out this life puzzle, some of us will find guidance in various therapies or other modalities to help us reprogram unhealthy patterns that we have acquired along the way. We will search for answers to some of life's key questions, such as: *Who am I? What is my purpose here? And what is the meaning of life itself?* The journey and answers are going to be different for each person.

It wasn't until my late 40s that I realized that as different as I was from my parents, I was still living my life based on some of their old stereotypical views. I was brought up believing that to be of value in the world, I had to be successful, have a title, and earn a lot of money. However, I learned that did not equate to sustainable happiness. I still didn't know who I was on the inside or how to find that lasting fulfillment in my heart.

While goals and accomplishments are fundamental skills, and esteemable acts build character, I found them to simply be lessons in my quest to get to know myself and find the answers to these reflective questions.

The things that helped me find that greater understanding of the meaning of life and how to cultivate and nurture a deeper relationship with my true "Self" included actively participating in various spiritual communities and programs including Alanon, Adult Children of Alcoholics (ACA), in, and having a daily disciplined practice of meditation. Of course, there were also many other teachers along the way as well.

I went from living in an unconscious state of survival mode filled with anxiety and fear (searching for my parents' idea of happiness) to learning how to feed my emotional spirit through developing healthier relationships with all facets of life, including death.

Midlife — the 50s and beyond — is a transitional time of truth and discovery where we come to a crossroads that will determine what the last chapter of this journey will look and feel like. This second half of life can be viewed or experienced as either a time of overwhelm and breakdown (the classic "midlife crisis") or discovery and breakthrough – a midlife awakening, utilizing our wisdom of the past as we embrace the excitement of our future.

Chip Conley, a modern elder and author of *Wisdom @ Work*, describes this phase of transition from mastery into mentorship as a time of human metamorphosis as we learn to shift from our ego-based thinking to the resonance of our heart and soul more deeply. It's a form of regeneration, embracing our elderhood with a new perspective of possibility, paving an extended purposeful path forward ... rather than falling into society's negative stigma – viewing retirement and aging as a devaluation or downside to life – the myth.

When we reflect on the evolution of a butterfly, it does present similarities to our human life cycle. A larva hatches from an egg; it instinctively nourishes itself until it reaches its caterpillar adulthood, when it finds a place to safely rest to spin a protective chrysalis around its body or pupa, completing its first cycle. It remains in this gestation cocoon, undergoing a remarkable transformation until it's complete, eventually emerging as a beautiful butterfly. Conley suggests that midlife is the gooey cocoon stage as we transition into elderhood. (Kübler-Ross has a different symbolic comparison to the butterfly in her book *On Life After Death*.)

For me, this transformation has proved to be an amazing, surprising gift and, overall, fulfilling time. I feel like I am an emerging elder moving into my butterfly phase ... I never imagined that I would be living in nature's abundant picturesque landscapes, finding thriving mature adult communities, and sub-teaching Tai Chi classes as part of my daily routine.

Now that I am past midlife, and into what I refer to as the wisdom phase, I truly understand the importance of striving to maintain this state of consciousness in all that I do. And to know that each phase of this sacred journey will play a part in my ever-changing identity as I continue to grow and learn how to love and be loved and enjoy this great gift of life to its full potential.

The Similarities Between
"Birthing & Dying" — "Babies & Those in Transition"

The birthing process is much like the dying process, and if you plan for both of them consciously, you will hopefully have a better chance of an intentional result. And if not — it's probably just part of a bigger plan directed by a higher source, overriding our ego-based ideas of how it should all go.

Some similarities between entering the physical world and leaving it begin with laboring. The mother labors in the birthing process, as does the infant coming into the world, as does the dying person working to get out of their body. A laboring woman's breath becomes rapid, and she sometimes needs help to focus and slow down its rhythm. Those in transition may also experience a shift in their breathing patterns and commonly require some coaching, reassurance, or even a relaxant from a hospice worker or practitioner.

We are sustained by our first breath and released through our last vanishing breath. Sometimes newborns arrive not yet fully circulated and may have a blue hue to their skin (depending on their ethnicity or skin color) from this lack of circulation throughout the body. This scenario also applies to some people as they leave their bodies — their extremities may turn blue (or discolored) as their organs shut down and their circulation begins to slow. Infants and those in transition both (usually) wear diapers, need to be carried or wheeled around, fed, and have their needs met by someone else. They both require a lot of unconditional love, guidance, compassion, and nurturing and deserve to feel a sense of safety.

"Death is not waiting for us at the end of a long road. Death is always with us, in the marrow of every passing moment. She is the secret teacher hiding in plain sight. She helps us to discover what matters most."
~ *Frank Ostaseski*[5]

Consciously Preparing for Death

What if you knew that today would be the last day of your life? Would you spend time worrying about it or live each moment to the fullest? What would you do, and with whom? What if you lived every day of the rest of your life as if it were your last?

As we come full circle in our conversation about the cycle of life, hopefully, you understand why preparing for death is equally important as preparing for birth. And that you will plan for it accordingly, with intention.

If we are blessed to live a long life or end up having a terminal illness, there is a bit more predictability to the timing of our death. While we'll never truly know what death is like (until we die) or when this moment will arrive, wouldn't it be nice if our loved ones knew how they could best serve and support our needs and spiritual preferences for a peaceful passage home?

As discussed previously, the first step to preparing for death is acknowledging its inevitability. The second step is making friends with the fear of dying. Once you have come to terms with those two things, you can think about the logistics of what comes next.

---

[5] Ostaseski, F. (2017) The Five Invitations: Discovering What Death Can Teach Us About Living Fully. New York: Flatiron Books. Quote reprinted with permission from the author.

Several fundamental details go into this process of preparation — legal, logistical, and spiritual. You'll find more information about these different aspects in Chapter 5, "Creating A Death Plan. For this section, I'd like to focus on the gift of having our needs met with compassion from the perspective of mindfully honoring the spirit of our soul as we prepare for completion.

I have supported several of these smooth transitions over the years, and I can honestly say that those who had their needs met and made peace with dying had a sense of tranquility about them as they crossed over. I pray that mine will be equally as gentle.

Being of service to people in their last phase has taught me so much about unconditional love. It has opened my heart to one of the most healing exercises of forgiveness, compassion, honesty, intimacy, and love. It has also given me great forethought into how I would want to spend my last months or days and formulate a vision for myself.

What would you want the end of your life to look like if given the choice? Even though this might be a difficult thing to think about or an uncomfortable conversation to have with your loved ones, it could also be one of the most valuable things you could do for yourself and them.

A few stories that demonstrate the benefits of planning mindfully and that offer a lovely perspective of leaving on our own terms are expressed in an interview I did with my then-94-year-old friend Florrie Shaun, as well as "Driving Miss Norma" and Nora Ephron's "exit" file, also found in "Creating A Death Plan."

Perhaps theirs and other stories in this book will inspire you to think about how to be there for others, as well as what you might intentionally want for yourself. My experiences have mostly been with adults, but I'd like to share a short story from an interview I did with Nancy and James Chuda about their daughter Collette.

The Chudas lost their daughter Collette to a rare form of cancer at the young age of five. While their loss was devastatingly painful, I found their story a beautiful example of acceptance that inspired me to look at death in a new way.

In March of 1991, after exhausting all options to help Collette fight her cancer, the Chudas surrendered to the inevitability of her death and embraced its reality with courage. Knowing that her time was coming to a close, they decided to have a beautiful end-of-life Easter party for Colette and invited everyone she had ever known — including her young friends. They colored hundreds of Easter eggs and spent the day celebrating her.

This act of love gave Collette and all of her friends and family a reciprocal way of letting each other know their impact on one another's lives while she was still alive. This gave everyone a sense of gratitude and completion as they walked her home together.

That interview introduced me to the idea that death could be experienced as a sacred and loving process by honoring the person in transition rather than something to fear. I found myself inspired by their story because it was such a courageous, beautiful act of love. When I left their house that day, I took with me a profound gift about death that I carry with me to this day and continue to pass along to others — that death is simply a transition from one dimension to another — a journey into the unknown — and something that can be celebrated.

A Soul's Journey Home:
Where Do We Go When We Die?

As a human's soul prepares to leave its physical body, one common thread I've seen is that they all engage in a beautiful dance between the two realms — the material world and the spiritual dimension — as they begin connecting to the spirit beings who came to support them with their integration process preparing for the other side. These integral interactions occur, off and on, over days, weeks, or in some cases months.

When I witnessed people transitioning between the two realms, some were aware of the process and would share their insights with me. Others would just include me in the conversation with their invisible friends, unaware of the two dimensions (which you'll hear about in the stories). My father described the spirit beings as very helpful and reassuring, giving him a sense of comfort and safety about his journey home.

I have also seen transitioning souls sent back to this dimension by those greeting them, presumably to complete another part of their karmic lesson(s) before eventually being released back to spirit. They had some fascinating (*verified*) stories about hovering between the material and spirit worlds, including seeing and hearing everything people were saying or doing simultaneously and dimensionally — and in several locations. Their stories gave me additional insights into what happens to some souls while dying.

I believe it is in this place of suspension — between space and form — that our spiritual communication is bridged, helping us receive messages and interact with their souls after they are gone. After the death of each of those I assisted, I could feel their energy around me and continued communicating with them. This connection is still present today and delights me when it happens randomly. Some people will feel this presence, while others won't. I am not sure why some are more available to recognize it.

I have witnessed some extraordinary things (that some might see as coincidences) around this continuum of a soul's existence through various communications both in my life as well as in the lives of others. Depending on the released soul's earthly personality traits, or the receptiveness of the living person on the receiving end, these messages can come through in either subtle or bold ways — sometimes funny, other times magical — and usually when we least expect them.

I think of their spirits as angels of consciousness that keep an eye on things for us from the spiritual realm. And I see their communication between the two dimensions as either little gifts of gratitude or important guidance. They are both a wonderful reminder that our loved ones are still very present in our lives and a positive affirmation that there truly is a continuum beyond our physical existence — as you'll see from the stories in Chapter 10, "Messages from Beyond". (These spirits have all helped me write this book.)

In some traditions, people leave the window open in a room of the dying and believe it aids the souls' transition into the next world. It is also a way of respecting and honoring the moment … a gesture of freeing the soul, letting go, and letting in; bringing in the fresh air from the outside world, and the promise of a new day and rebirth.

Ultimately, death is simply the completion of one's lessons in this life cycle. When the body falls away there is an expansiveness of spirit. The soul is then released and freed to move about in the cosmos doing angelic things until it evolves into the next incarnation or level of existence or nonexistence — again, depending on your belief. The essence of our loved ones' soul's consciousness as we have known them in physical form lives on and is always with us in its purest form of love, protecting and guiding us.

SWEET PAULA
A LESSON OF COMPASSION

Vignette Four

Paula, my stepsister, was unique; as I've mentioned, she had special needs. Our relationship was very challenging, yet it was one of the most important of my life. She taught me great lessons about many things, especially compassion and unconditional love.

I met Paula when I was about six years old when she was in her early 20s. Again, as I've mentioned, I didn't care much for Rose, so I didn't particularly want to meet her daughter but that's what was happening on that Sunday morning during my weekly visitation with my dad.

I sat on my front porch steps waiting for the three of them to arrive. I found the perfect seat where I could see them coming up the walkway. As they rounded the corner, Paula was lagging behind. She was a fairly large young woman, awkward in her gait, distracted, and displayed mannerisms I had never seen before — not what I expected as a potential playmate.

My best friend Lexy lived next door, and her cat routinely perched on the steps watching everyone. When Paula saw the cat, she got so excited that she let out a screech that could have shattered glass. It scared everyone, including the cat. Rose tried to contain Paula's over-enthusiasm and hold her back from charging the frightened animal but was unsuccessful. Fortunately, the cat escaped unharmed. I found her enormous energy very overwhelming.

I had never been exposed to this odd behavior and certainly never taught how to interact with people with special needs. Paula lived on a ranch run by nuns outside of Los Angeles, so I was relieved that I didn't have to see her very often. The doctors had inappropriately labeled Paula "retarded."

When my father married Rose, Paula officially became my stepsister. My dad was a kind man and saw something in Paula that others hadn't recognized — that she was capable of much more than anyone assumed. Together he and Rose decided to bring her home to Los Angeles.

They found a great living situation for Paula at a semi-assisted home in the Fairfax area where she had her own room and could come and go as she pleased. Once she got settled, my father began teaching her necessary life skills. He taught her how to take a bus, do laundry, and shop for incidentals, which eventually empowered her to live on her own in a small apartment in West Hollywood.

When I went to live with Dad and Rose, Paula became a problem for me. In my early teens, if I wanted to go out with my friends, the condition was always that I had to take Paula with me — to the skating rink, to the beach, everywhere. It was a lot to expect from a grieving, dysfunctional teen.

Paula was always so volatile and impatient that I began responding to her by mirroring her behavior back to her. Eventually, my friends confronted me about how I was treating her and taught me how to respond differently, with more patience and kindness. Still, I secretly resented my stepsister.

Rose & Paula — Mother & Daughter

It turned out that I wasn't the only one who had a hard time with Paula's behavior: Rose didn't understand her either. She spent much of her time yelling at Paula and belittling her for not behaving the way she wanted. They fought constantly, yet when Rose found herself disabled, they ended up spending most of their days together hanging out at the Farmer's Market, a landmark destination in the heart of Los Angeles.

Over the years, Paula became somewhat of a celebrity there as well as in the outlying neighborhoods. She knew the shopkeepers, bus drivers, elderly people, kids, the bankers — everyone. If you paid attention to Paula, she would do anything for you. Depending on their patience level and personality makeup, people either loved or dismissed her.

Her parting words to people were always, *"May the angels fly with you."*

Changing Times: Who's Watching Paula?

After our parents passed, I became responsible for watching over Paula and her companion bird (who mimicked her behavior of yelling). I never imagined that I'd be caring for the woman who had been such a thorn in my side for all those years!

Three months after Rose died, I had a major horse accident and could barely care for myself or my daughter, so taking care of Paula was not a consideration. During that time, Paula developed a blood disease that required extra oversight, and one of my cousins and his wife were able to facilitate her treatment, which eventually brought her into remission. We were lucky that despite Paula's disabilities, she could always find someone to help her when she needed it.

My Awakening

Since Paula appeared to be doing well after I recovered from my accident, I went on to create and produce a show that consumed most of my time for many years. Once I finished that project and spent more time with Paula, I realized how neglectful I had been. The truth was she really wasn't capable of efficiently caring for herself.

By then, Paula had a variety of other problems, including rotted teeth, excessive drooling, and a condition that caused her to doze off during a conversation. Her balance was off, and she had several nasty falls, where she suffered, among other things, a severe injury to her hand. Her ring finger was so badly infected and swollen that I had to take her to a jeweler to cut off her mother's wedding ring.

When Paula couldn't tell me exactly when she had fallen, I understood that she had no real connection to her body or time. I saw a child in an adult's body that had survived my absence with the help of her guardian angels.

In that "aha" moment, I realized that Paula had many of the same characteristics and behaviors I had seen in the kids I worked with on the spectrum. Was it possible that Paula had autism? It all began to make sense, and that's when I decided to take a more active role in Paula's care.

After investigating her problems of drooling and dozing off, I learned Paula's doctor had misdiagnosed her autistic behavior as manic depression and prescribed lithium. She had been on it for several years.

Over the next six months, I weaned her off the lithium and had her teeth fixed. The drooling decreased as I reduced her dosage, and her mood began to stabilize. Paula had a lifelong weight problem, but once she had new teeth and I taught her how to make more nutritious meals for herself, she was able to maintain a steady, healthy weight. That gave her more self-confidence and happiness than she ever had before.

A Sisterly Rhythm & Subtle Changes

Paula and I got into a steady routine until 2014 when I began to notice subtle changes in Paula's coordination, mental health, and behavior. Keeping her apartment clean was more difficult, telling time was challenging, and the accidents were more frequent. I decided to teach Paula how to use a cane. At first, she was reluctant, but once she saw that it gave her more control over her body, she adapted nicely and even gave the cane a name: Gabriel. She referred to it as her best friend.

Then one weekend, when I was out of town for Mother's Day, a dog attacked Paula — mauling her non-dominant hand. He broke her middle finger, which required a splint, and she needed stitches in all four fingers and her thumb.

I returned home the next day and found Paula in bed with a high temperature and blood everywhere. Several stitches had broken open because she lacked the coordination necessary to care for herself with one hand. I rushed her to the hospital, where they admitted her for ten days due to complications from her injuries.

When Paula was released from the hospital, she needed extra care, so I assembled an incredible team of caregivers she adored. I felt great relief, but it was short-lived because I received a call from a panicked Paula the following night telling me she couldn't breathe.

I called 911, and Paula was readmitted to the hospital, where she almost died from septic pneumonia.

The doctors told me Paula's blood disease had returned, and her organs were shutting down. They also feared she might have experienced significant brain damage and weren't sure if she'd be able to walk again. This was terrible news for Paula because her whole existence revolved around her independence, social life, and ability to care for herself. I knew that if she lost those things, her quality of life would be bleak. Paula spent the next two months in the hospital, where she gained 60 pounds and was bedridden.

A Singing Buddha

Eventually, Paula rallied, and we needed to find a suitable rehabilitation facility. Our cousin Nancy came into town to help me. We only had 48 hours to find a place to move Paula because the hospital needed her bed. The first center we visited was dark and cramped, and the residents appeared depressed and unhappy. It was not a good experience or fit for Paula.

We truly needed a miracle for Paula and asked the universe for guidance in finding a happy place with a Buddha and a fountain. We also asked Rose and my father to assist us from the other side by showing us a sign so we would know it was the right place.

The next place we visited was very different, and we knew our luck had changed. The front door opened onto a bright, wide entryway, and while Nancy went to inquire about the facility, I was drawn to the main dining room, where live music was playing.

When the person singing walked by the doorway, I quickly grabbed Nancy's arm to show her what I saw. To my surprise, it was an Elvis impersonator. Nancy and I both knew that Elvis Presley was Paula's Buddha. When Paula was young and home visiting her mom at work cutting hair at the hotel, she disappeared for a few minutes, only to return with the real Elvis Presley holding her hand.

He was staying at the hotel, and Paula had captured his heart with her unique ways. She asked him if he'd come to meet her mommy, and he agreed. That moment was one of the greatest thrills of her life. Being such a sweet person, not only did Elvis go with her, but he also let Rose cut his sideburns. So YES, Elvis is Paula's Buddha.

There were also several other signs of affirmation that this was the right place for Paula, including a large cage with singing birds. It was as if Rose and Dad were right there with us orchestrating some divine intervention.

Once we got Paula settled into the facility, the reality of her physical and emotional condition hit her hard. Her two biggest fears had come true — she was overweight again and unable to walk. It was painful to witness, but I did my best to help her adapt.

Over the following five months, Paula had several other emergencies requiring additional hospital stays that were very traumatizing and took a toll on her mental and physical health. Consequently, in November, everyone involved with Paula's care decided she would no longer be transferred to the hospital for medical treatment.

Her chart preference was changed to read, "Make patient comfortable and call the doctor for an in-house assessment moving forward. Do not transfer to the hospital." Paula happily agreed with this arrangement.

I visited Paula several times weekly to make sure she had everything she needed. During this time, we had several intimate conversations about our sisterly relationship. We reminisced about the challenges and the memorable moments that made us laugh. She also expressed her gratitude in her unique childlike way for all I had helped her with over the years.

Synchronicity & Divine Timing

As we approached Christmas, it was time to find a new permanent assisted living arrangement that would be her final destination. I found a perfect place with a beautiful garden, a fountain, and two lovely patios on a tree-lined street close to my house. Paula was upbeat and excited, which made me happy. All we needed now was for a room to become available.

Knowing she wouldn't return to her apartment, Paula and I agreed that it was time to pack up her things and close that chapter. Other than her sentimental items and necessities, I gave everything away. All her belongings went to residents in her apartment building who were in need. It gave us great pleasure knowing what a difference Paula's things made in their lives.

I left a picture of Paula on the shelf above her gas fireplace and said a prayer of gratitude for giving her a safe space for more than 30 years before closing the door one last time. When I arrived home, a message on my answering machine confirmed Paula's acceptance into her new residence. Paula was elated at the prospect of having a private room again.

The days leading up to Christmas were spent finalizing details for Paula and preparing for a work-related trip to Hawaii. On the morning of December 24th, I called the center to confirm the time of their holiday party, but when the owner answered the phone, he began apologizing to me. I had no idea what he was talking about and asked him to slow down and tell me what happened. He finally revealed Paula was back in the hospital, despite the "Do Not Transfer" order in her file.

At first, I was livid, but I quickly remembered something that I always tell my clients: Everything happens exactly how it's supposed to happen. As I drove over the hill to the hospital, I kept repeating my mantra: Everything is in divine order and exactly as it should be.

The Three Spirits of Christmas Greet Paula

A petite nurse named Arlene greeted me when I arrived at the hospital. I quickly explained the mistake and that there was also supposed to be a "Do Not Resuscitate" order in Paula's file. Arlene had just been transferred back to the main hospital after serving in hospice for years and understood my concerns. She told me she would put a "test refusal" order in place until the doctor arrived — a bold move on her part.

In doing this work with those preparing to die, I am always amazed by the subtle signals we are given from the universe — Arlene is the name of Paula's favorite relative, who had passed away a few years earlier. When I mentioned that to the nurse, she looked me in the eyes and said, "It was meant to be. There are no accidents."

I didn't know it at the time, but that was my first sign that Paula was actually preparing for her transition.

Paula was awake and alert when I got there and apologized, hoping I wasn't mad at her. I told her not to worry and that everything would be okay. Moments later, her body started failing. Alarms went off, and nurses ran into the room and began resuscitating her despite my efforts to tell them Paula had a DNR order, which no one could find.

They worked on her frantically, and I realized there was nothing I could say or do to stop them. Just then, I felt Paula's energy standing next to me, laughing and telling me to sit down and witness the chaos. And so, I did. It was an odd feeling. Shortly after, they succeeded in bringing her back to consciousness. She and I had one last beautiful, intimate conversation about our journey together before she closed her eyes and dozed off.

What a blessing.

The doctor arrived a few hours later and told me that the best thing we could do for her was to keep her in the hospital and bring hospice in to help with her transition. I agreed but told him that I'd be leaving in two days for a week. He said she probably would pass during that week, which I had already suspected.

There really wasn't anything else for me to do that would have contributed to Paula's comfort or process, so I moved forward with my out-of-town commitment. The doctor and I put a plan in place, and before leaving, I kissed Paula's forehead and told her I'd be back later. She smiled.

I took care of some pre-trip details and picked up my friend Debbie, who loved Paula. We headed back to the hospital, where we met her new nurse Abraham whom I had spoken with earlier that evening via phone. Debbie and I both took note and commented on his name in relation to it being Christmas Eve and giggled.

Most of Paula's hospitalizations were horrible experiences, but this time was different. It was quiet and peaceful. Her room was dimly lit and had a beautiful view of the Hollywood hills, *including her old apartment*. Soft music was playing, and I felt such a sense of serenity. She was no longer hooked up to monitors. All was calm. I stroked Paula's head, and Debbie and I prayed for her to have a smooth transition. She didn't open her eyes during that visit, but we certainly felt her love in the room.

Debbie and I left the hospital and stopped at a universal church on our way home to pray for Paula and give thanks for her in our lives. We arrived towards the end of the service in time to hear the angelic voices of the choir. At the end of the performance, the chapel went dark, leaving one candle burning, representing the dawn of life.

Each of us had been given a candle when we arrived. The first candle was lit and used to light the next person's candle, and so on, until every candle in the church was aflame. Debbie and I cried as we sang Christmas carols. The candles lit up the faces of each person, highlighting the tapestry of family histories of all ages and ethnic backgrounds. We walked out of the chapel emanating light on that Christmas Eve. It was a magical experience.

An Apology & Saying Goodbye

On Christmas morning, I got a call from Paula's best friend, Morna, insisting she needed to visit Paula at the hospital. I agreed. She arrived mid-morning to an alert and fairly coherent Paula, and they were able to share laughter along with a song and one last conversation about their fond memories. Morna called me when she left and said she loved her friend and would miss Paula.

I arrived at the hospital around 2:00 p.m. and met Russ, Paula's day nurse. When he told me his name, I laughed and said that it was the name of my father's last attendant. I then realized Paula's three nurses were possibly a sign of communication from the other side from the three most influential people in Paula's life (her mother, my father, and cousin Arlene), all of whom were happily there to assist in guiding her home.

Paula was restless when I got there, but she never opened her eyes. I snuggled her face with her soft stuffed panda bear. As mentioned in earlier stories, people usually wait for a specific thing to feel complete, but I still needed to figure out what Paula was waiting for.

When I turned inward for guidance, I got the message that she was waiting for me to handle one piece of unfinished business from our childhood: an apology for how I had treated her in my teen years by not letting her sit with my friends and me on the bus.

That cruel act was something that had always bothered me as an adult. While this completion was more for me than for her, I believe it healed some deeper karmic stuff between us. I expressed how sorry I was for my behavior and asked for her forgiveness. She squeezed my hand in acknowledgment. At that moment, I knew we had come full circle.

Once I had made amends, I told her she was a good girl and how proud I was of her in response to her always saying, "I was a good girl today. Aren't you proud of me?"

Her words always meant that she hadn't fought with anyone during the day and had followed all the rules.

Since Paula had always waited for instructions from me, I gave her permission to let go of her body. I assured her that it was no longer serving her and reminded her that I would be leaving in two days and would not be seeing her again in this life. I gave her two options: the freedom to leave while I was still there or after I went. It was entirely up to her. I told her how much I loved her and how grateful I was that she was my sister, and it was time for her to let go and let God guide her home.

Russ came back into the room just as I was getting ready to leave, and I told him I believed that she would be transitioning on his shift. He walked over and touched her body, and replied, "I don't think so. Her circulation is still normal, and her vitals are relatively strong."

I reaffirmed my thought that all the signs (including that my father's last caregiver's name was also Russ) suggested she was going to take my cue and make her transition.

It was tough to leave the hospital that day, knowing that would be the last time I would see her in this lifetime. Saying goodbye to a loved one's physical body can be surreal. Each of us finds our way of doing it.

I leaned in and kissed her forehead. I prayed and said, "Thank you. Thank you. Thank you. I love you. I love you. I love you! Now it's your turn; may the angels fly with you." I left the hospital, asking the universe to support her gentle passage.

Once in the car, I called Debbie to update her. Out of respect for the holiday, I didn't feel comfortable calling anyone else on Christmas Day, but Debbie had been part of the process over the last few days, and it gave me a sense of relief that I could call a friend.

Debbie invited me to stop by for dinner on my way home, and since she lived around the corner, I did. We finished dinner at 4:55 pm, which I noted on a wall clock behind her head. I expressed my appreciation for her lovely meal and then excused myself. As I pulled into my driveway, my cell phone rang. It was Russ. Paula had taken her last breath, and her physical body was at peace. She made her transition home on December 25, 2015, at 4:55 p.m.

I burst into tears and immediately began talking to her, letting her know what a good girl she was and how proud I was of her for being able to let go.

Paula's presence and gifts continue on today from the spirit world and often surprise me, forever reminding me of her wonderful sense of humor and innocent love. (Please see Chapter 10, "Messages from Beyond".)

CHAPTER 5

CREATING A DEATH PLAN

Three Women Prepared
for the End-of-Life on Their Terms

The following stories are three delightful examples of people who had that important conversation with their friends and family and were able to have their final wishes fulfilled.

Driving Miss Norma: *Living Life With, No Regrets*

Ninety-year-old Norma Bauerschmidt and her husband, Leo, had been married for over 67 years when he died of cancer in 2015. Her remaining family included their son, Tim, his wife, Rami, and their 12-year-old Standard Poodle, Ringo.

Norma's kids had retired early and given up their more traditional lifestyle to travel around the country in their recreational vehicle. When Leo was moved into hospice, they came home to help support their parents.

Within days of Leo's passing, Norma was diagnosed with stage four uterus cancer. After assessing their mom's health and living situation, Tim and Rami knew she couldn't live independently and invited her to join them on the road. At first, Norma was reluctant;

however, when her doctor presented her with the typical treatment options — surgery, radiation, and chemotherapy — she did a quick check-in with her kids and was able to respond with confidence, "I am 90 years old; Ringo and I are hitting the road." The doctor thought it was a great idea.

That was the day Norma said yes to an amazing adventure traveling across the country — a road trip that her family dubbed, *Driving Miss Norma & Travels with Ringo*. Her decision to live the rest of her life enjoying quality time with her loved ones turned out to be the best medicine anyone could have prescribed.

The following 14 months were an incredible journey as they all got to know each other in a whole new way, enjoying an unexpected deeper level of closeness. Miss Norma got to do things she had never done before, like taking a hot-air balloon ride, riding a horse, walking on the beach, and visiting numerous national parks and treasures — Mt. Rushmore, the Grand Canyon, the Rocky Mountains, and Disney World among others — all while indulging in as much beer and cake as she wanted. Their time together was filled with laughter, joy, fun, and unconditional love, and it was an invaluable gift for them all.

When Norma's needs became more than Tim and Ramie could handle on their own, they contacted a local hospital, where they were met with full support from the staff on all levels, physically, emotionally, and spiritually.

In the end, Norma transitioned comfortably on her terms while in her own bed in the RV. Everyone was at peace with the outcome and felt a deep sense of completion by being part of her entire process. With love and kindness in their hearts, Tim, Ramie, Ringo, and a host of others all walked Norma home in such a beautiful way.

Ringo eventually joined Norma six years later, and I imagine she happily greeted her faithful friend with a smile.

Special thanks to the Bauerschmidt family (and Ringo) for allowing us to share their inspiring story of living life to its fullest with no regrets. You can read all about their adventures on their website, MissNorma.com.

Florence Anne Shaen: *Attitude, Humor & Love*

Florrie was a spirited woman whom I had the pleasure of knowing for over 30 years. She was the aunt of one of my dear friends, and up until 2020, we would routinely have dinner on Sunday nights with various family members who happened to be in town. I always enjoyed listening to her entertaining stories told with quick-witted humor.

One evening, shortly before Florrie's 80th birthday, she invited me to come and check out her latest "real estate investment" at Westwood Village Memorial Park. Greeting each other at the cemetery, we watched as a squirrel ran by, and I playfully said, "Oh look, they even have wildlife here." Florrie added, "And dead life too."

We both laughed, and then she told me her marker would read: "Attitude, Humor, and Love." What a perfect epitaph.

As we walked through the cemetery, Florrie shared how her views on death had changed.

"I have feared death all my life, as I believe most people do. However, since I bought this space for myself here at Westwood

Village, I have a much better sense of acceptance about dying. I have a plan, a weird type of enthusiasm for where I will go — a beautiful, peaceful environment where everyone is happy. Not that I am in any hurry to get there.

We should all be excited about where we are going to end up. This place is quiet, small, intimate, and full of life. My ashes will be placed in a little niche in a private gated garden. A small vase will be filled daily with fresh flowers, and there is a bench for my family and friends to sit on when they visit. The park is also non-sectarian, so everyone is welcome.

The people here are just delightful, and they will take care of everything. If I die while traveling, they will ensure I get home safely. I was fortunate to get a spot right below one of my best friends. I feel like I'm in divine company here with several of my dear friends who have already passed and celebrities such as Marilyn Monroe, Hugh Heffner, Natalie Wood, Rodney Dangerfield, and Truman Capote."

"Let's face it, Florrie, you will always live in an upscale neighborhood," I said.

Florrie nodded in vigorous approval. After all, she had lived a fabulously full life. It was her belief that when our bodies are done, they are done — and we can't change that — it's just part of life.

That said, as we left the cemetery, Florrie implored me, "Please make sure I'm breathlessly dead before they put me in the oven for cremation. Do a mirror test!" I assured her I'd take care of that last request for her.

When I asked Florrie if she wanted all of her ashes placed in her sacred niche in the garden, she said, "No, not all of them. I have asked my niece in New York to take a small offering of my ashes to sprinkle on Broadway — because then I'll have made it on Broadway."

Florrie passed away in August 2023 from natural causes. I had planned to visit her at the end of August, but unfortunately, my plans changed. When I told Florrie I wouldn't be coming, she expressed great disappointment. She called me several times over the next 24 hours to confirm that I was no longer coming. I didn't realize it then, but perhaps that was what Florrie was waiting for to feel complete.

The following day, her body began to shut down, and Florrie was transferred to the hospital, where she remained in transition for another few weeks. It was a bit of a bumpy ride, but in the end, I was able to help walk Florrie home over the phone and tell her the words she needed to hear to let go. She was surrounded by her loved ones.

Nora Ephron's "Exit" Plan

Nora Ephron, the noted journalist, writer, and filmmaker (*When Harry Met Sally*, *Sleepless in Seattle*, *You've Got Mail*) left nothing to chance when creating her death plan. She outlined every detail about her memorial service and titled it "A Gathering for Nora," which she left in a file labeled "Exit."

Ephron knew that by doing so, her family could orchestrate her vision with no questions about what she would have wanted. There were even instructions with a list of names of whom she wanted to speak, in what order, and where she wanted the service held — the

Lincoln Center's Alice Tully Hall in New York City. Her efficiently crafted plan made things much easier for her family and friends during their time of grief, making it a true celebration of Ephron's life — like being at a fabulous Hollywood party.

Creating Your Plan
Three Elements: Legal, Logistical & Sentimental

I think the two hardest parts about devising a death plan are thinking about it and discussing it with a loved one. Shortly after my parents passed away, I had a serious horse accident, which was a big wake-up call. What would have happened to my daughter and assets if I had become incapacitated that day or worse, had died? I suddenly realized that everything I had worked so hard to create could have been lost or misdirected in that split second. Who would have financially cared for my daughter or my special needs stepsister? Being the sole provider for two other human beings and a business owner was a huge responsibility.

Since most people don't like to talk about death, preparing for these life-changing situations often gets overlooked. During my recovery period, I came to terms with the vulnerability of my affairs. I devised a plan to appropriately take care of all of those I was responsible for if something unexpectedly happened to me. It has, of course, changed over the years, and I make sure to keep it current.

While creating that plan, I faced two uncomfortable yet crucial conversations — one with my friends about the "what ifs," and the other with myself about my deeper fears around death itself.

Beyond the legal details and logistics of my affairs, I also started thinking about the other elements of what happens when we die, prompting questions about my wishes and what I would want someone to know about me.

Outlining these things might feel weird at first, but the truth is we never really know when our time will be up. Whether you care about these details or not, consider this: your plan will make things easier for your loved ones by giving them guidance during a difficult and disorienting time of grief.

The following details are essential to consider:

- Make a list of all of your accounts (banks, credit cards, social media, etc.) and passwords, along with any essential legal documents, and let a trusted loved one (or two) know where that list can be found upon your death.
- If you have assets or are responsible for someone else, what type of legal plan do you have in place — a will, trust (i.e., a revocable or irrevocable living trust), a Do Not Resuscitate (DNR) order, medical directive, and durable power of attorney specific to your state?
- If you knew when you would die, how would you like to spend your final months/days?
- How do you envision things going after you die? Would you like to have a hand in creating your funeral, wake, or celebration of life? What would you want it to be like if you threw one last party for yourself? (For example, I have told both my daughter and good friends to honor me in nature with a spiritual ceremony and then throw a fabulous [sober] dance party outdoors somewhere they know I'd love.)
- Is there anyone, in particular, you'd want to see, make amends to, deliver some gratitude, or resolve a situation to

feel complete? (This is kind of a trick question; if you can clean up old karma, you should consider doing it now and not waiting for your deathbed.)

- Are you an organ donor? If so, do your loved ones know?
- What would you like done with your remains? There are many options beyond traditional burial or (fire-based) cremation, like being "planted' or "mixed into the soil" under a tree, cremated by water, or composted, among other environmentally friendly options. Explore the pros and cons of each process (economic, environmental impact, etc.) to decide which option aligns best with your beliefs and desires. And if you don't really care, let those closest to you know that as well.
- If you choose a more traditional burial, where do you want to be laid to rest, and who will pay for it? This is a costly endeavor and something you might want to take care of while alive.
- If you choose cremation (or one of the alternatives), where do you want your ashes scattered or buried? Do you want them spread on land, water, or at a special place — maybe several? When I traveled, I took a little bit of my father's ashes and put them in some of his favorite places on the road and around town. My dear friend Dave wanted some of his ashes sprinkled in my yard. (More about Dave in Vignette Five.) You can also have ashes made into a piece of glass or jewelry.
- Instead of flowers at your funeral or celebration of life, do you want donations to go to your favorite charity? If so, identify it (or them).
- Would you like to leave a friend something special not outlined in your will or trust? Write it out or give the item to them before you are gone.

- Playing music at the end of life can be very soothing for those in palliative care or transition. What type of music would you like to hear? It could be your favorite artists and tunes or something soothing, meditative, or Music-thanatology, a clinical modality designed specifically to support the dying.
- If none of this truly matters to you, then tell your loved ones so they won't wonder what you might have wanted.
- And, on the flip side, it would be nice to know certain things about your friend or family member if you are their primary support person and will be helping with or handling their affairs. These are all simple questions we rarely talk about or ask.

Last But Not Least …

Who will care for you in that last phase of life? There are many different options, including hospice care, a death midwife or doula, a family member, or private nurses — although it is usually a combination of people who work as a team.

To be clear, here's the difference between hospice care and a death midwife or doula:

- Hospice care is a program to support people with less than six months to live when curative treatment is no longer a viable option. It focuses on a patient's emotional wellness, comfort, and pain management (administering medication) in their final days. A doctor can order it for implementation in their home, an assisted living facility, a nursing home, or a hospital.
- A death midwife or doula is a person who assists in the dying process by tending to the terminal client's needs to help them

feel safe, comfortable, and complete throughout their transition, much like the birthing process.

Both hospice care and death midwives/doulas supply emotional, physical, and spiritual support to the patient and their families and help usher them home in a compassionate and loving environment.

For example, my father's team consisted of his physician, myself as a liaison and decision-maker and death midwife/doula, a private in-home care nurse to do the heavy lifting and night care, and a hospice team to manage his medications and ensure his comfort. I called them the angels of mercy. They were such a gift.

Another important question to ask yourself is do you want to die at home or in a hospital? Both my father and stepmother spent time in the hospital before I brought them home, where they would be more comfortable in familiar surroundings. Keep in mind that outlining your preferences in a death plan doesn't always mean that's what will happen; it simply means those are your wishes. Sometimes, a spontaneous decision must be made based on the immediate situation and resources.

Relatedly, depending on where you live and if you're dealing with a terminal illness (feeling hopeless and in a lot of pain), you might want to take matters into your own hands and consider physician-assisted dying or aid-in-dying. First publicized by the controversial work of Dr. Kevorkian, a pathologist who helped over a hundred people take their own lives through what was called assisted suicide.

There are currently at least ten states that have "Death with Dignity" laws in place to support a compassionate end of life. There are also facilities or destinations in the world where people can go to die on their terms, for example, the Kashi Labh Mukti Bhawan guest house in Varanasi, India.

For more information about how to put together a death care directive, contact an estate planning attorney, a healthcare social worker, hospital staff, or other reliable professionals. In this chapter's Resource section, you'll find additional educational sites to help you do your homework. No matter your age, now is the time to start putting your affairs in order because you never know when that moment of departure will happen. You can always make changes over time that reflect your new ideas and circumstances.

DAVE'S PEACEFUL DEATH

Vignette Five

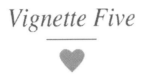

Soulmates, Trusted Love,
Karmic Ties & Saying Goodbye

Dave, AKA "Luke the Drifter," was a humble and gentle man passionate about many things — music, reading, traveling, trains, photography, architecture, wearing hats, and walking in nature. He walked every day of his life, no matter what the weather was like, until the end. Dave was a musician and a lawyer and served his community.

I met Dave during my senior year of high school. I still remember the first time I saw him. It was love at first sight — a deep familiar love, something you can't explain — and an inner knowing of many lifetimes together. He had beautiful blue eyes, full kissable lips, and long dark wavy hair. My heart was his at that moment and forever.

Over the years, our relationship shifted and changed as we grew together and on our separate paths. Our first chapter reflected the innocence of young love, where your legs go weak, and you get that flutter in your chest every time you see each other. However, nine months later, that phase was cut short when he moved back to his hometown on the East Coast. I don't remember why he left, but I was heartbroken.

Fortunately, we were able to maintain our friendship by writing letters to each other. They were few and far between, but I received each one with that same warm and fuzzy feeling inside. To this day, I still have every picture he sent me. He was always in my heart.

To my surprise, Dave returned a few years later to make California his new home. I was already involved with another man at that time, but I was able to arrange a place for him to stay across the street from where I was living in Nichols Canyon. I would cook dinner for everyone a few times a week, and Dave and I would have breakfast on the weekends. That gave him a stable base while he looked for a job and apartment, and it was wonderful to have him close again!

Even though the stars hadn't aligned for us romantically, I always invited Dave to holiday dinners, birthday parties, and even both of my weddings. He later walked me through those divorces and stood by me at my loved one's funerals. He was part of my family and very involved with my daughter, Danielle. He attended all her activities — sports, plays, and musical gigs. I eventually asked him to be her godfather.

When Danielle got married, Dave was in the wedding ceremony, standing right next to her biological father. The two men remained lifelong good friends. Dave was my best male friend and taught me about trust and the true meaning of friendship and unconditional love. He supported Danielle and me in everything we did.

After living in his small apartment for over 25 years, Dave bought his first house in 2001. It was a Craftsman bungalow in the heart of Hollywood that had been destroyed in a fire. His mission was to restore it to its original form, which he did, paying close attention to every detail, Dave later named it "Hummingbird Ranch." It was his pride and joy and was featured in an architectural magazine.

After the passing of both of my parents, Dave and I once again found ourselves attracted to each other on a romantic level. While we both had valid concerns about what might happen to our friendship if things didn't work out, we were willing to take the risk.

This was an exhilarating time of discovery as we embarked on exploring new adventures together — romantic getaways, restaurants, live music, and festivals. We were independent people with varied interests who had been single for many years, so having a partner opened up a whole new world for us as a couple. Things weren't always perfect, and there was a lot of compromising because we were both fairly set in our ways. However, our relationship gave us great lessons in communication and intimacy as we learned how to support each other's needs in a new way and still be true to ourselves.

We continued that intimate relationship for the next ten years. At that point, we began growing in different directions again and mutually agreed to redefine our roles, moving back into our best friend status. We did this with much gratitude for the years we spent together as a couple, and thankfully, we were able to forever remain each other's voice of reason and loving support.

Shortly after that decision, Dave developed a debilitating case of pneumonia which lasted more than a month. He never fully recovered his full strength or weight after that but was able to carry on over the next decade, living a full life — occasionally traveling and continuing his community work.

In 2020 when the Covid pandemic hit, Dave, like everyone else, had become isolated, restricted, deprived of socialization, and consumed by the fear of the unknown. We spoke daily during this time, but it was almost two years before we finally met again in person. Those two years in lockdown took their toll on Dave's health; he lost more weight and had trouble breathing. Seeing him gave me a clearer perspective of his emotional and physical abilities. My heart sank as I felt him slipping away.

While Dave was in denial about his health and had no interest in seeing a doctor, he finally admitted that keeping up with the responsibility of homeownership was becoming more difficult for him. Every time we spoke, he would mention his struggle, so eventually, I suggested that maybe it was time to sell the house. Dave refused for a long time, but when his father was nearing his end of life, he finally gave in.

Dave's plan was to help his dad, who lived in Florida, and once he was gone, move back East to be near his sister, Sue, and her family. I believe, on some level, Dave knew how sick he was and that it was in his best interest. Unfortunately, his father passed away before he could get there, but thanks to modern technology, Dave was able to be with him and his sister when he took his last breath, which gave him a sense of completion.

Once the house sold, I helped Dave close up Hummingbird Ranch, and he stayed with me for a few days before heading east. We took one last walk together on our favorite trail in Franklin Canyon, something we had done together for over forty years, before saying our final goodbyes. When I took him to the airport, I knew in my heart that would be the last time I would see him. It was a bittersweet moment of emotion as we lovingly held each other, but I knew Sue would take good care of him.

Despite everyone's concerns about Dave buying another house when he was so weak, he did. I believe he just wanted his own space where he could have his belongings around him in the comforts of his home to meet his end on his terms. It proved to be his last project.

The house was down the street from his sister, which afforded them the opportunity to walk every day and routinely share meals. In the evenings, they would sit on her back porch sipping mojito cocktails and eating fresh peach ice cream. He also spent time with her husband, children, and grandchildren, who enjoyed the gift of getting to know "Holly Dave" (short for Hollywood).

Sue eventually talked Dave into seeing a doctor, who told him he had advanced Pulmonary Fibrosis, a progressive lung disease. In his case, it was a terminal diagnosis, and the doctor predicted Dave would have another year at most.

Dave had studied many philosophies in his lifetime, from the bible to Buddhism, and he was comfortable in his beliefs about death. He also loved to know how things worked, so he began reading everything he could about the spiritual and material aspects of death and dying. I believe this helped him in the process of orchestrating his own gentle death. He would share some of his discoveries with me, which, in turn, gave me insight into how I could best support him daily from afar.

I asked Dave if he wanted Danielle and me to visit him one last time, but he said no. I understood; we had spent the last four decades with him, and now it was his biological family's turn. They were all so grateful to spend that last year with Dave, which made him happy.

However, Dave and I continued our daily conversations where we would reminisce about the different phases of our love and adventures, talk about death, and express our gratitude for each other.

During that last year of Dave's life, I also decided to sell my house and start a new chapter in the Midwest near my daughter and her father. One of the first things I did was buy two deck chairs and send Dave pictures of them so he would know there was always a place for him to come and sit with me at my new house. We also continued our Sunday evening game nights on Zoom, where the rest of his West Coast family (all now in the Midwest) had a chance to spend time with him and bring him up to date on their lives. That was the one thing he asked us to continue throughout.

Danielle also extensively talked with Dave about his life, their relationship, and his process of dying in those last few months. It was a beautiful, intimate experience between godfather and goddaughter in their completion cycle — something she will always cherish.

As he neared the end, there were several things that Dave was waiting for — not to feel complete, but rather so he wouldn't be a burden or ruin someone else's day or plans with his passing. That's just who Dave was. Yet, with a family of that size, something was always happening — a birthday, sports event, planned vacation, holiday, etc., so finding the right time wasn't easy for him.

As Dave's breathing became more labored (and I would imagine painful — even though he never complained) and he got weaker, it was time to implement his end-of-life plan. He turned 71 in May, and his sister's birthday was in June. Given the circumstances, Dave finally decided that he would be ready to go after her party on the second Saturday in June.

He and his sister met with hospice to discuss the details, and then the timeframe was left in his hands. I had left Dave a few messages that week, but he never returned my calls. I thought perhaps he was having phone issues, but I now know he simply didn't want to talk to me yet about his decision.

On the night of Sue's birthday party, I had also been at a party in my neighborhood. When I was walking home, as I approached my house, to my surprise, I was greeted by something I had never seen before growing up in California: an abundance of fireflies dancing like fairies in my front yard.

I immediately unfolded the chair I was carrying and sat down to watch the show for 45 minutes. After a while, I realized the dancing fairies were only in my yard — it was as if they were sent to me as a gift. I was mesmerized by the magical moment and wanted to share the experience with Dave right away. I tried to call him while sitting there, but he still wasn't answering. I figured I would tell him about it the next day when I saw him at our Sunday Zoom gathering.

Dave arrived on Zoom looking frailer than usual and asked us about our week first. I immediately told him about the fairies in the garden, and he smiled from ear to ear, sharing my joy. After hearing all of our stories, Dave's tone changed, and he became emotional. He then told us that this would be our last time together and that he had made arrangements to begin hospice care.

Dave explained that he had already eaten his last meal before our gathering and would be turning off his phone that night. I wanted to support his decision, but it was so abrupt that I couldn't help but ask him if we might speak privately one last time the following day. The gamut of emotions that ran through my mind and physical sensations were so overwhelming that I couldn't breathe, yet I was so grateful when I heard him quietly say "yes."

Even though we knew this day would come, none of us were emotionally prepared for the reality of the moment. Our hearts were broken knowing this would be the last time we would see him. We could all see that it was equally as difficult for him to say goodbye to us, as we were saying goodbye to him. I wasn't sure how to respond, but later that night, I wrote Dave one last text and prayed he would read it.

"Thank you for sharing this lifetime with me. Your love and generosity of spirit are forever infused and imprinted in my heart and soul. You have been an amazing friend, lover, godfather, and so much more to me. I am so grateful for our time together and how you've always been there for Danielle and me. You are my true love, and I love you more than words could ever express. Sweet dreams, my friend, as you embark on your next adventure ... the great mystery. The fairies are dancing in my garden tonight, and their magic will always remind me of you. I will be here listening for your whispering words of wisdom in the wind and trees ... and in nature all around me on my walks. I am forever grateful for you in my life. xoxo"

Later, I found out that everyone else from our Zoom group had texted him as well. I can only imagine how overwhelming it must have been for him. I didn't get much sleep that night, and my tears of sadness and gratitude continued throughout the morning. I finally composed myself a bit and decided to call him after lunch. It rang for a long time before his niece finally answered. She said she was spending time with him while her mother took care of a few last-minute details before returning to be with him.

Dave was sleeping, but when he heard my voice, he opened his eyes and said he wanted to talk to me. His niece put us on speakerphone, and I began to cry again when I heard his voice. I told him how much I loved him and that I would be lying next to him if I were there. Dave quietly agreed and affirmed he had read my text. I made one last request: to be the beneficiary of his favorite hat. He said he thought that could be arranged, and we both said our final goodbyes as best we could — after all, we were both bidding farewell to our soulmate.

Sue and one of her daughters sat with Dave throughout the night, rereading all the texts he had received as he rested comfortably. Eventually, they dozed off until around 1:30 a.m. when the ladies were awakened by Dave yelling "Sue!" over and over.

When Sue gently asked, "What, Dave?" he joyfully exclaimed, "Good morning, Sue!" And then he drifted back off into a relaxed deep sleep again. He had said those words to her every morning for the past year ... a daily ritual that lifted both their spirits and that she loved.

There was a delightful summer rain drumming on the roof that morning, and Sue later told me she could hear the long rumbling of thunder off in the distance. It was gray outside, so the room remained dark even as the day began to break.

In the end, Sue was alone with him when she noticed his eyes were looking upward toward the corner of the room. There appeared to be light shining in his wide-open, crystal-clear eyes — the whites so bright and the blue, iridescent. Sue sensed that her brother was looking at something quite magnificent.

Sue moved closer to him and said, "I think it will be easier than you think, Dave. Can you see Mom, Dad, our old dog Trixie? They are just over the hill with Jesus. Do you see them? Run and jump into the everlasting arms of Jesus, Dave, and he will carry you the rest of the way and say, "'*Well done, thou good and faithful servant.*'"

With that, Dave took his last breath and was released from his physical body into whatever awaited him.

Dave's Parting Gift

As Sue witnessed Dave's final moments on her end, I was also having a magical experience. As fate would have it, my contractor, Don, was scheduled to install my new carpet that morning. When he arrived, I explained that one of my best friends was in transition, and I was unusually emotional. He expressed kind words of condolences for the situation.

Don began preparing the meditation library room floor, where he had just removed the old carpets and was getting ready to cut the new materials. I quietly sat in the living room, observing the chaos of the moved furniture and thinking about Dave. Suddenly I felt this wave of inspiration move through me, and I was guided to find my colorful artist chalk somewhere in the misplaced bookcases. I found them and began drawing affirmations, pictures, and words of gratitude on the bare wooden floorboards (half-covered in black felt) awaiting the new coverings.

The words and symbols flowed out of me like a river of creativity. Tears of joy ran down my face as I expressed my love for Dave and our blessed journey together. It was an energetic experience beyond words.

At one point, Don came in and said, "Oh my, I'm going to take a break because I don't want to interfere with whatever is going on here with my weird energy." We both laughed, and I thanked him.

Once the floor was completely filled with color, gratitude, love, and the magnificent vibration of light, I felt complete and returned to my chair in the living room. Moments later, still basking in the energy with a deep sense of inner peace, I received a text from Sue telling me that Dave had just passed. I felt in my heart that my inspiration was an aspect of Dave's release from our physical world and that he had made it through the veil of dimension and was safely home.

"Power and healing can be found in our grieving — intentionally and purposefully with others." ~ Kathy Arnos

A Different Type of Grief …

I had grieved many times before Dave, but this time was different. With my other relatives, my grief had been suppressed. First, with my mother because of the secrecy surrounding her cancer and the silence that remained after her death. There was no conversation about her passing or acknowledgment of my emotions. Consequently, I was taught to stuff my feelings and that there was shame in those feelings.

I was afraid if people knew how scared, sad, and broken I felt that I would be sent away like Paula was when she was young. I had no idea what type of behavior was acceptable or normal. There was no guidance, tools, compassion, or nurturing love to be found, thus no time to grieve within the web of my extreme fear.

My experience with my father was my first opportunity to consciously explore the depth of spiritual relationships and death and better understand the process of dying and completion. Our journey together taught me how to listen, the importance of completion, the integration process, and how to be of service.

However, in the end, there was no time to officially grieve my dad's passing either because I had so many other responsibilities, including straightening out his affairs, organizing care for Rose and Paula, running my business, and caring for my daughter. Yes, I was able to honor him in the labyrinth and at the celebration of life that his AA buddies threw at Roxbury Park, but I had very little time or privacy to absorb the gravity of my loss.

Dave was very similar to my dad in many ways — his Zen-like personality, ability to forgive and love unconditionally, ethics, and even some of his mannerisms, like how they both knocked on things and whistled while they walked. Neither of them liked deep conversations about their feelings, and I could count on one hand the number of times I saw either of them get outwardly angry. The similarities stopped at how it felt to say goodbye to each other on this physical plane.

Mourning a parent vs. mourning a partner/soulmate/friend is quite different. I had shared all levels of myself with Dave — physical, emotional, and spiritual. He was also the first loved one whose physical needs and affairs I wasn't responsible for during and after his death.

This time it was simply about the knowledge of the process and witnessing a beautifully orchestrated, peaceful death. There were no excuses … there was plenty of time to finally experience a healthy grieving process. It's a gift to feel every emotion — the highs and lows — in a loving, supportive, honest, open environment. I held space for my process as each thought arrived and declined invitations to participate in any activities that might be too overwhelming. It was the first time I truly acknowledged my limits and abilities.

I looked through pictures and danced to our favorite songs with tears of sadness and joy for our journey together. We set a place for Dave at Thanksgiving with a picture in his spot with his happy hat perched on the top of his chair. We filled his glass with sparkling water to toast his energetic presence. I spent many hours texting and talking to his sister and my daughter sharing our feelings.

Also, many unexpected feelings showed up over the next nine months, like guilt over my not being more patient and emotionally available in our romantic relationship. These are character defects that I am still learning about myself today. I had so many stories swirling around in my mind about how I could have done things differently. Over time, I learned these thoughts and feelings were all normal and common.

Fortunately, through my meditation practice and amazing support team, I was able to reconnect to the present moment, process those feelings, and remember the truth about consciousness and who I am as a human. In the end, we are all simply pure consciousness and unconditional love — doing the best we can.

Everything is in divine order — today — and always, I have complete peace with any lingering grief. When it shows up, I feel the feelings and marvel at the joys of our beautiful relationship.

Letting go and embracing the opportunity to learn how to honor the true nature of the dimensional aspects of our relationships is a gift. And I am so grateful that I could grieve healthily this time and experience that precious opportunity.

I feel Dave's presence in every moment of every day — he continues to surprise and shower me with magical blessings daily. Dave also has a wildly quirky sense of humor and often makes me laugh.

I also have a small heart urn necklace with an amethyst crystal and stone that hangs from a lamp on my desk with Dave's ashes. I find comfort in knowing he is not only spiritually always with me but that a small tangible part of him is also near helping me write these pages. His light continues to shine brightly.

CHAPTER 6

WRITING A LIVING EULOGY

A eulogy is a speech or piece of writing that acknowledges the importance of the life lived and reminds survivors of the memories and legacy left behind. It is something that is typically given after someone has died. A living eulogy is simply expressing those sentiments while they are still alive.

I have found that writing a "note of gratitude" or receiving one from a friend or family member is always a lovely exchange of energy. When you think about it, a eulogy for someone is simply an extended version of this thank you note where you acknowledge that person before they die, for the gifts they have given you and their role in your life — however small or large, loving or complicated that relationship has been.

As I have become more connected to the precious element of life, my interactions with friends and family members have changed. With each conversation or visit, I try to remember to exercise my gratitude muscle and convey how much I cherish that friendship. We never know when that might be our last conversation, so it's crucial we let people know how we feel about them. While I am complete in most of my relationships, a few people have slipped away or were taken unexpectedly. I wish I had had one of those conversations with them or had written them a note of gratitude while I had that opportunity.

A few years ago, I read a heartwarming story about a man who practiced Buddhism and was dying of cancer. His family and friends were very much a part of his care during his transitional process. One of the things they asked his friends to do during this time was write him a living eulogy. While some read their words to him directly, others left notes with the family to be read to him privately. This type of intimacy was a beautiful way of completion for everyone.

The family also posted a sign to visitors at the door that read, "Bring Only Joy," respecting the importance of creating a loving environment to support the process of him leaving his physical body in a way that honored his Buddhist faith. This sentiment also encouraged his positive rebirth to wherever his soul's experience would take him. Both of these actions are a lovely idea.

This story teaches us how writing a living eulogy lets us put our thoughts together more intentionally. By taking time to reflect on the uniqueness of that relationship over time rather than trying to express your feelings in a vanishing moment, can bring a greater sense of connectedness to that relationship — whether for an hour, a day, a year, or ten years.

If none of these ideas or thoughts resonate with you, perhaps just spending time with your friend talking or listening will be the perfect way for the two of you to feel complete. These ideas are simply here to plant seeds about connecting with people in ways you might not ordinarily think about doing.

No matter how your reflection is delivered — written, verbalized, or simply by listening and at whatever phase of life you deliver it — it will be perfect. I find I do it differently with each relationship, and it always brings a special moment of connection and love.

Some ideas for what your living eulogy can include:

- A gratitude list
- A list of the qualities that you most admire about them
- A detailed description of how they have impacted your life
- Your thoughts about a special event or a shared experience
- Your insights from a specific lesson or trade you've learned from them
- Or being, that we never know when that day will arrive, throwing a party or living funeral at any age where people deliver messages of gratitude to the honored guest over a meal

Not All Eulogies Will Be a Note of Gratitude

Not all relationships inspire a love note. There are as many hard karmic lessons in the world (filled with anger and resentment) as healthy ones. Family dynamics can be complicated and challenging, so writing a heartfelt eulogy when a person you struggle with is alive may be difficult.

Ideally, it would be wonderful if we could all work through our resentments while our loved ones are still living, but I couldn't do that with my stepmother. The one thing I was able to do while caring for her in those final months was to find some compassion for her brokenness. Thankfully, that compassion inspired my last words to her: "I love you." And strangely, I meant it. It was as if all of the resentment of the past seemed to merge with the pure essence of love in that exchange, even if it was only for that moment.

After her passing, I struggled to find a fond memory or some loving thoughts to share in her eulogy. After all, she had raised me with such unrecognizable love and anger. My words were few and gracious — all I could honestly say was that I was grateful for the many lessons she had taught me.

It wasn't until years later, after doing significant inner spiritual work, that I found forgiveness and acceptance for my stepmother (and myself, for my part) and our dysfunctional relationship. I finally recognized that she did the best she could with suddenly being thrust into the parental role of a grieving teenager. I also realized that forgiving her didn't mean that her behavior was okay or my feelings weren't valid; it simply meant that I wasn't willing to carry that anger and pain around in my heart anymore.

This awareness gave me a better insight and understanding of my anger and how my resentment blocked me from being connected to my own heart and learning about the true essence of love. When my inner child began to heal, I could appreciate my stepmother's role in my life and realize how grateful I was for everything she had done for me — which was so much.

Moving into that place of acceptance and forgiveness was a big relief. I only wish I could have come to both of these things while Rose was alive, but as most of us know, we come to our awareness and healing when we do, and not a minute sooner. (See Vignette Three, My Stepmother Rose: *Finding Forgiveness & Healing Resentments Through Acts of Service.*)

I want to leave you with one more story if you ever have to write a eulogy for one of those more complex relationships. My friend Kate told me how writing and delivering her father's eulogy was a defining, pivotal moment:

"The eulogy was a moment of total healing for me. For the most part, my dad and I did not have a close relationship, but my efforts

to work on myself and to forgive a lot of what I viewed as his indifference toward me — my whole life — meant I could give a eulogy to his 'aspirational self.' I talked about the man I knew he wanted to be, who did his best as both a father and a friend, and I meant every word. I didn't have to embellish at all. Also, I was able to make it humorous and light in parts because that was who he was. That moment was transcendent for me. While speaking about him in the saddest surroundings of all time, I was able to laugh. And, so did other people."

JOHN: MR. WIZARD'S GIFTS

Vignette Six

My journey with John was about the reciprocal nature of giving and receiving unconditionally with deep gratitude — a relationship without expectations. I learned new insights about the completion process and how to support someone passing with grace, ensuring their dignity remains intact — a simple act of kindness with love and humor — that can profoundly impact a transitioning soul. John's gifts of appreciation filled my heart with love.

John was a technology guru and cutting-edge energy healer with a great sense of humor. People called him "Mr. Wizard" or "Jedi" at his memorial celebration. Others simply called him the "Woo Woo Man." He could wave his hands and shift negative energy in minutes, inexplicably helping people heal from physical and emotional illnesses.

I met John when he helped my (then) five-year-old daughter find relief from a severe case of whooping cough using energy work and light therapy. He was an unusual man, and I wasn't sure what to make of him at first.

A motorcycle and race car enthusiast, John had spent most of his younger years working in the studio prop department, eventually owning his own prop company. He could build anything and had a genius-like fascination with electricity and light. He went on to create several unique light and electronic healing devices.

When a Healer Needs Healing

While John was extremely talented at healing others, he didn't take good care of himself. He was a heavy smoker and liked to indulge in unhealthy foods. He had his first stroke in 2006 and another a few years later.

The next time I saw John after this second stroke, his physical condition had declined considerably, and he needed a cane and human assistance to get around —something he navigated with a sense of humor. Then in 2012, when John was diagnosed with bladder cancer, his wife, Yolanda, decided to cut off all communication with their friends. I am not sure why, but it was very disheartening for all of us.

John's Last Chapter

Two years later, I received an unexpected call from Yolanda letting me know that John was in a nursing home and inviting me to come and visit him. I was excited to have this opportunity to reconnect with him and prayed that the universe would support me in having time alone with him.

The facility was a bright and quiet one-story building in Burbank, not too far from where they lived. When I walked in, I didn't have to ask where John was because I could hear Yolanda's gruff voice vibrating in the hall. She was pushing John in a wheelchair down the hall with her back to me, so I walked up behind her and asked if she needed help. It took her a few minutes to recognize me, which gave me a good insight into the toll her act of service had taken on her. Thankfully, John knew who I was immediately and was elated to see me.

The three of us walked out to a patio area where John was to be served lunch. We talked for about 45 minutes before Yolanda grew impatient and went to find out where their food was. I was happy to have those few minutes alone with John and used the time wisely.

I told him how much I appreciated him and all of his help over the years. I thanked him for his kindness in always treating my family even when we couldn't afford it. John's speech was slow, and he was having trouble connecting his words to his thoughts, but his eyes conveyed that he was taking in every word of what I was saying. The two of us held hands and began to cry. I knew then that John wasn't long for this world and that it might be the last time I would see him. At least now he knew how grateful I was for our friendship and his generosity.

Yolanda returned a few minutes later with an attendant close behind with their lunches. John tried to feed himself but was having trouble, so I helped him while Yolanda ate her lunch. She was clearly exhausted from caring for him for many years.

Before leaving, I took a few pictures of John and one of the two of them for my memory book and told them to call me if they needed anything. I left that afternoon with a full heart and feeling complete in our relationship. It was a wonderful visit.

Moving Into Transition

The next time I heard from Yolanda was several weeks later, a few days after Christmas. She let me know that she had brought John home, and he was now in full transition. She also told me he was extremely uncomfortable; she didn't know what to do for him and needed my help.

I told her I'd be there the next day. When I hung up, I meditated and (telepathically) asked John what he was waiting for. He answered immediately and expressed that he was waiting for two things: He needed Yolanda to have a plan for her future, and, from a karmic point of view, he intended to usher in the New Year before leaving this body. I called Yolanda back, and she agreed to put together a plan so that we could tell John about it when I got there.

When I arrived the next day, Yolanda greeted me and took me into their small dining room, which was now the central gathering place. The room was hot and cramped, and John was in a bed by the front window wearing nothing but a diaper. A kind Asian caregiver was sitting across from me, ready to assist with any of John's needs, and two elderly dogs were taking up much of the floor space. The scene was odd, considering they had a large three-bedroom house.

Some people preparing to lose a loved one will create a womb-like environment to feel safe and comfortable, which I felt was clearly the case here. It had only been a few weeks since I last saw John, yet he was almost unrecognizable. He was visually and emotionally already on the other side, just waiting for confirmation that Yolanda had a plan so he'd know she'd be okay once he was gone.

I spoke to John softly, acknowledging his process before sitting down with the caregiver and Yolanda. I explained that he was straddling both worlds and trying to leave his body, which was why he was so restless.

John was visibly uncomfortable as he tried to navigate the sheets to find a soft spot for his bony body. Yolanda and I spoke to him about her plan for a few minutes from our chairs, and then I got up and went over to John and leaned in so I could engage with his eyes. I wanted to see if I could get him to connect to our physical dimension one last time, despite the discomfort he was experiencing leaving his body.

Using my normal voice, I called his name, and he opened his eyes. I told him Yolanda's plan and had her come closer to connect with him and express anything else she wanted to say. She embraced the moment and began to cry, reassuring him she would be okay and that it was time for him to let go. I told him how much I loved and appreciated him and said that we would make his journey a little more comfortable. John nodded in gratitude.

Once that bit of business was complete, I asked Yolanda to bring me a pair of his favorite undies and a t-shirt. She returned with a Ghostbusters t-shirt, a sure sign that John was already orchestrating things from the other side with his wit and sense of humor. I asked for a pair of scissors to cut the shirt up the back, and then I slipped it on from the front with the emblem intact. We then cut a piece of diaper off a pull-up and put it inside his undies to give him a little more comfort and dignity. He was now appropriately dressed for his journey.

I proceeded to do Reiki on him to help him relax, and he settled nicely. That was the last interaction John had with this world. He rested comfortably for the next few days while waiting for 2015 to arrive.

John's Humor & Appreciation from the Other Side

On New Year's Day, I headed up the coast to meet a friend for breakfast in Malibu before taking our annual hike. It was one of those mornings when things just weren't going my way, so when my friend, who was usually very generous, decided to claim both of the heart-shaped rocks we found on our hike, I felt a bit resentful. I can usually shake off these feelings, but on this particular day, I was having trouble.

After the hike, as I drove away, I thought wouldn't it be nice to start this day over again? I decided to head down the coast to one of my other favorite spots, a place that I refer to as my private beach, where I frequently go to meditate and enjoy a "wave" vacation. Very few people know about this public beach.

When I arrived, there were only a handful of residents peacefully meandering around the shore — I was grateful for the opportunity to start my day over. As I made my way down to the water, my foot hit a palm-sized rock in the sand. I looked down and saw it was a heart rock. It felt like a message from God reminding me that I was loved.

It was perfect.

I picked up my treasure with a big smile and continued down the beach. I had only gone about ten feet when I spotted another heart-shaped rock. I sang out, "I hear you, Spirit. I know I'm loved, and there is plenty of love to go around."

Things became quite magical that New Year's Day: every few feet I walked, another heart rock appeared. I found 16 heart rocks throughout my walk and shared some of them with various strangers — couples in love. It was an extraordinary experience to both receive and freely give away these gifts of love from nature.

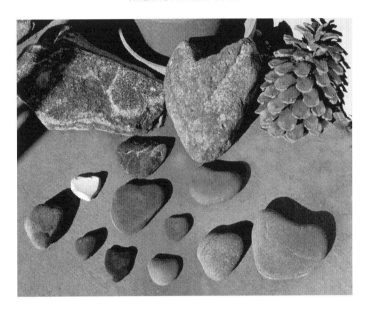

When I got home that afternoon, there was a message from Yolanda telling me that John had died. When I called her back, she seemed at peace with his passing and had already planned for John's memorial service the following Friday.

The celebration was simple and sweet, and it was interesting to learn more about John's history — we know very little about each other when it comes down to it. When I walked into the church, I was glad to see one of our mutual comedian friends Rick, and to swap stories about John. As we were walking to the gravesite, my foot hit something in the grass. When I looked down, I found it was a heart rock.

I burst out laughing as I connected the heart rocks on New Year's Day and John's passing. I told Rick the story and asked if he thought I should put this new heart rock on John's casket.

He replied, "There are plenty of rocks where John is going. This is another gift for you," and we both laughed.

Thank you, Mr. Wizard, for your gifts of love and appreciation — keep waving those hands and making magic happen, even from beyond. I think of you often.

CHAPTER 7

A CELEBRATION OF LIFE

The truth is, there is no right or wrong way to celebrate someone's life. While the person's character and the circumstances surrounding their death will often dictate the tone of the ceremony, almost any type of memorial service is appropriate or acceptable today.

Depending on the situation, a celebration of life can either take place while the person is still alive — in the case of terminal illness — or after they are gone. Celebrating a loved one while they are still here is similar to the principles of a living eulogy, where you can actually voice your thoughts of gratitude. For instance, as mentioned earlier in Chapter 4, when the Chudas threw a beautiful goodbye party for their young daughter, Collette, that proved to be a wonderful day of completion filled with love — for everyone. In essence, they threw her a "living funeral," which is becoming trendy as people are more accepting of the idea that death truly is an essential aspect of life.

Another example of a living funeral was one that marked a milestone occasion: *Death Over Dinner* founder, Michael Hebb's 40th birthday. His friends, who playfully refer to him as 'the death guy,' threw him a living funeral while he was very much alive and healthy (with no end in sight). They told "Michael stories" and also spoke about others they loved who had passed away. Rather than a morbid occasion, it was filled with heartfelt love, some laughs and tears, and, most importantly, provided attendees with an opportunity to be vulnerable and open while making peace with mortality.

That said, traditionally, people have followed the standards set ages ago by their religion, spiritual practice, or culture in honoring their loved ones. This is usually done in a specific timeframe as a stand-alone event with a formal funeral, wake, or memorial service at a religious or cultural place of worship.

However, while writing this book and speaking with a wide range of people from different backgrounds, I have noticed that some of the younger generations are now beginning to question these older traditions, and families are more open and flexible to making changes based on their specific needs.

For example, a Jewish friend in her 50s admitted that she had decided not to do the final graveside ceremony dictated by tradition called an "unveiling." It's technically the ceremonial dedication of the memorial marker or headstone, but it's really a ritual that is more for the bereaved than the decedent. It's intended to end the formal mourning period and give family and close friends one more opportunity to face their loss and affirm their commitment to living and life itself.

Nevertheless, the logistics of the ceremony were daunting — her mother was buried on the East Coast, and she and her dad lived in California. There was no doubt the trip would take a significant physical toll on her infirm father, and my friend also was worried about the impact of the long journey and caretaking tasks on her.

After some discussion and taking time to process their feelings (mainly guilt, but also sadness) around breaking this important custom, they agreed that they could say the traditional prayers remotely from California with the help of an East Coast relative who volunteered to attend graveside and "Zoom" them in. Thus, they found their way to a suitable compromise and embraced a modern version of this traditional practice of completion.

Another example is a story about the sudden death of an Irish man whose six daughters, when planning his funeral, decided to break the tradition of men carrying the coffin. As the strong women the father had raised, they decided they wanted to be the ones to carry him from his house to the church and the graveyard and lower him into the ground. Some of their local faith leaders and family members vehemently objected to their decision, but the women were defiant. They asserted it was the best way to stand with their father in death — a part of their Irish tradition — and honor his life. And, so they did ... holding him at shoulder height throughout.

These types of deviations are happening with different faiths worldwide. I have also found that more and more people of all beliefs and across generations are moving away from the old models and adopting new approaches to honoring their loved ones with different ceremonies — simply dubbing them a *"Celebration of Life."*

People are embracing more of a relaxed upbeat experience that can be done anytime, anywhere, that allows them to design a service in a way that honors that person's true spirit within their social communities — aspects that some family members might not even know about them. This type of gathering has more of a party atmosphere and focuses on the joy the deceased brought into their lives rather than the sadness of their death. Some families will do both — similar to a wedding and reception, a formal service, and then a party atmosphere.

I have attended a variety of these different types of services over the years in churches, temples, and synagogues, as well as those of the

Native American culture on sacred land, meditators in community groups, and even atheists and agnostics. I've especially enjoyed the non-traditional ones in various locales: at sea, in a summer garden, in a park, on an island, in studios, and even in a local retail store … just about anywhere. Some were elaborate, while others were very simple. No matter where or how the event takes place, they are all considered a celebration of life.

A few things to remember when planning for the day is that it is to commemorate the memory and aliveness of that person and their life — what they were passionate about, their favorite foods, their hobbies, your experiences with them, their accomplishments, their service to others, what they were all about, and who they were as unique individuals — a reflection of their true essence.

This ritual is also for us as we begin our healing process. A place to come together in community with one another, to show our love and appreciation to someone who has touched our hearts in some way. For some, it's about making peace with the loss, a sense of closure, an acknowledgment that one phase has been completed — a form of saying goodbye that can act as a transitional moment of moving forward, beginning a new chapter.

I am often amazed that, inevitably, I will learn new things about someone at each service. When Dave died, and his sister Sue was planning his service, I realized that there were aspects to him that I didn't know. For instance, he had a deep connection to the Bible, as she included some of his favorite scriptures in the ceremony. I found it quite surprising, considering how close we were. I believe Sue felt the same way about certain things I knew.

There are so many sides to each of us, with so many complexities: the side our family knows, how our friends view us, work colleagues, and other significant people in our lives. A Celebration of Life is a beautiful way to knit all the pieces together — the tapestry of our lives.

That is one of the main reasons I felt compelled to write the book — to start the conversation about our end-of-life care and death so we can know each other more intimately while we are still alive. I can't emphasize this enough — talk to your loved ones.

But many people don't have this conversation, and that's where I invite you to use your intuition and imagination, knowing that whatever you do will be the perfect send-off to celebrate their distinctive essence and life. The key is to show up for the moment and do your best with what you know.

The following are some examples of unique services that have honored the true essence of people I have loved. My intention is to plant seeds of creativity to encourage you to explore how you can authentically celebrate your loved ones when they are physically gone. I also encourage you to envision your own after-party and to share those thoughts with others, as Florrie Shaen, Norma Bauerschmidt, or Nora Ephron did in Chapter 5, "Creating a Death Plan."

My Father

My father was Jewish but didn't regularly attend religious services, and we never discussed his thoughts about his funeral. Since he was the first family member to go in my adult life, Rose and I agreed the perfect way to celebrate him would be to let his buddies in Alcoholics Anonymous put together his service. We felt it would represent his authentic nature and truly honor the love and appreciation my dad shared with all who would attend.

They rented the recreation room at the park, where they gathered weekly for 29 years and held a beautiful AA-type meeting in his honor. A few hundred attended, and an anonymous donor catered the whole event. I spoke about my father and what he meant to me through my affectionate tears while his friends told jokes about him being the treasurer for 29 years (off and on — because they trusted him). They also told stories about how he helped inspire them in their recovery and impacted their lives. It was a wonderful ceremony; we all felt him in the room with us on that warm summer day.

Although my father and stepmother had purchased burial plots years before their passing, in the end, they both changed their minds and opted for cremation. When you have someone's ashes, the question remains: what do you do with them? You can place them in a container somewhere in your house where their presence can watch over things, or you can set them free in nature at one of their favorite places.

My dad and I had joked about me traveling after he had passed and how I could take small pouches of his ashes with me and leave a little trail of him along the way. He liked that thought and felt that eventually, in a sense, we'd end up traveling the world together.

So, that's what I did for the first 15 years following his death. I even took some of them to a music festival in Colorado, one of the few places we had visited together in my teens. I could feel his joy right there with me — he loved to dance and listen to live music.

Seeding The Garden & Labyrinth: A Second Celebration of Life & Completion Ceremony

Sixteen years later, our traveling journey ended one Veteran's Day when my daughter, Danielle, her father, Tom, and her godfather, Dave, came over for brunch. It was the perfect day to celebrate my dad's memory again, as he had served in World War II — earning a Purple Heart and the President's Award, along with 12 other prestigious medals.

After our brunch in the garden, we took Daddy's ashes out to the labyrinth. Tom said a few words about my dad's humor before spontaneously reaching into the bag and grabbing a handful of his ashes. We all started belly laughing like little school kids and couldn't stop. Danielle and I viewed her father as prim and proper and couldn't believe what we saw. I think he even surprised himself — forever reminding us of my father's playful energy.

We took turns sprinkling his ashes along the path and in the labyrinth, delivering Daddy back to the earth as though we were seeding the garden.

The joy and laughter we experienced through this ceremony became an invaluable and treasured memory — a true celebration of our family's love. Today, I feel my dad's energy and voice all around me wherever I am. He is in the wind, the bird's song, the flutter of a hummingbird or butterfly's wings, and a blooming flower. He is everywhere, and I am never alone.

Rose

When my stepmother died, the only family left in California was her nephew, his wife, my stepsister, and myself. Her few close friends had died decades earlier. The only thing that had given her purpose in her last 20+ years was that she was the president of the homeowners' association where she and my father had lived for over 30 years. She always enjoyed running the show and being in charge — that is who she was.

I posted an invitation in the elevator of the building for her service, and a handful of residents attended. We sat around and joked about how Rose ran the building with a strict hand. We served lox, bagels, and cream cheese with coffee, which she would have enjoyed. It was short and sweet.

Bud Ekins

My friend Bud was a man of few words, and I never heard him speak about religion or his heritage. He was one of Hollywood's top stuntmen and a world-champion motocross winner who collected antique motorcycles and cars. He also owned a Triumph motorcycle dealership in the San Fernando Valley, affectionately known as "The Shop." Producers, directors, racers, actors, and motorcycle enthusiasts from around the world loved to come and hang out with Bud and the gang — you never knew who would be there.

His celebration of life took place on the Warner Brothers backlot in Burbank (CA), where hundreds of folks showed up riding motorcycles and driving antique cars. The family produced a lovely video of their life adventures with him and his incredible story, which they showed in a large screening room on the big screen.

Triumph honored him with a Special-Edition motorcycle, which was the envy of the group, and everyone wanted to capture a picture of themselves on it. Bud's memorial completely reflected a true representation of all aspects of him, and I'm certain he had a good time and was sporting one of his mischievous *Bud Ekins* smiles that I always cherished.

PAM: A GIFT FROM THE UNIVERSE

Vignette Seven

♥

What happens on the other side? Thanks to my friend Pam, I have some insights for you. Enjoy this amazing story — it's truly a gift and a miracle.

I met Pam, her husband Dave, and their twin girls, Danielle and Megan when they moved into the house on the corner of our Westside rental. Our girls were toddlers, and they looked and acted like triplets. Both of our Danielles were very spirited, and Pam and I became lifelong friends. She was a kind woman, vocal activist, conscious visionary, and an excellent teacher to me on living a healthier lifestyle.

Our neighborhood block party ended in 1987 when our families each bought homes in different areas. We continued to spend birthdays and special events together and would talk frequently via phone. Interestingly, Pam and I both went on to become writers and holistic practitioners who enjoyed connecting with like-minded people.

Pam later created a circle of women who would come together a few times a year to share our successes, sorrows, and lives with each other. We were mostly activists and natural healing enthusiasts passionate about empowering people through knowledge. She called us the Circle of Wise Women.

When Pam turned sixty, the Wise Women came together to celebrate her milestone. We showered her with our love, appreciation, and gifts, ate delicious food, and shared inspiring conversations.

An Unexpected Turn in Life

Shortly after that, Pam and I decided to set up a brunch date with our partners (both named Dave). We were to make a full day of it, but it didn't take long for me to realize that Pam wasn't feeling well. She had low energy, trouble breathing, swollen glands, and a sore throat. She explained that it had been going on for over a month, and nothing she tried had helped.

Pam scheduled an appointment with a Western physician for the following week to run some tests. Unfortunately, the tests identified that Pam had acute leukemia. Another piece of unexpected news that week came when her daughter Danielle announced that she and her longtime partner were expecting a baby. Both discoveries came as a complete surprise and were pivotal moments.

Before Pam could explore or investigate holistic or traditional treatment options, she developed a severe case of pneumonia. I received a call from Megan telling me that her mother had been admitted to the hospital because of complications from pneumonia.

When I arrived at the hospital, Pam was comfortable, sitting up and smiling, and we had a nice visit with the family. As we were leaving, Pam informed us that they would be transferring her to a different hospital in the morning, where they were better equipped to treat her specific type of leukemia.

Unfortunately, in the process of her transfer, things took a turn for the worse. Pam had a pulmonary hemorrhage that was potentially a result of her pneumonia treatment. The incident was physically and visually traumatic to her body, as well as the family members who witnessed it.

When I arrived at the new hospital the following morning, Pam was hemorrhaging from all openings in her body. She was in the ICU, where they had packed her nose with gauze to stop the bleeding, but it wasn't working. Pam was sitting up and conscious but very upset and scared. Her biggest concern was that she would bleed to death before Dave or the girls arrived. The attendants were preparing Pam for a transfusion, and given her concerns, I quickly asked the nurse what medications she was on. I was stunned to learn they were giving her a blood thinner and asked to speak with the doctor immediately.

The nurse returned a few minutes later and removed one of the IV bags. When I asked what she was doing, she said the doctor agreed that Pam no longer needed the blood thinner. Shortly after, a male nurse arrived with a blood bag for the transfusion. He hooked Pam up and walked away. As I was standing there, I glanced down and saw blood dripping onto the floor. I couldn't believe my eyes. There was a hole in the bottom of the bag, which meant that this precious life-saving blood was now potentially contaminated. I rang the alarm bell again, and they quickly replaced it with a new bag.

I'm not telling you about these hospital mishaps for any other reason than to emphasize the importance of a patient having an advocate when dealing with medical care. Nurses and doctors are human and equally as capable of making dangerous mistakes as providing life-saving actions.

When I returned the next day, Pam was in a quarantined ICU, unconscious, still hemorrhaging, and now hooked up to life support. Megan held her hand, talking to her while trying to make sense of the situation. Despite the doctor's and nurses' words of encouragement, they all felt the only thing that could save Pam's life would be a miracle.

Love and Prayers

Days passed, and our Wise Woman Circle continued to visit daily and hold prayer vigils. We did Reiki on her (an energy healing technique), envisioned her return to the family and our group, and infused her with our love and light energy. Yet, there were still no visual or physical changes. Several of us felt her presence in the room hovering overhead with little interest in returning to her body.

By the end of the second week, most of us felt hopeless and helpless. As a holistic practitioner, I believed there had to be something we could do; I just wasn't sure what it was. I spent the next day and night praying and meditating, looking for an answer.

The message I received was that we hadn't tried giving her one of the most common homeopathic trauma remedies to stop her bleeding. When the right homeopathic remedy is used, it can trigger the body's innate immune response and, in some cases, produce spontaneous results. The question was would her family be open to using it?

I returned to the hospital the next day with the remedy I thought best suited her situation in hand and spoke with Megan about her potentially giving it to Pam. She said, "I know my mom would want us to try it." After discussing the option with the rest of her family, it was unanimous - they would try it.

Later that day, Megan gently slipped the remedy into Pam's mouth, where it could safely melt between her lips and teeth. I believe she repeated the treatment a few times that day.

Pam's Miracle — A Gift from the Universe

Over the next eight hours, the bleeding stopped, and eventually, Pam opened her eyes. The miracle we prayed for happened — Pam had returned to her body! The doctors were shocked and amazed.

Over the next few days, it quickly became apparent that her will to live was back. Every day was a new lesson in patience, courage, and recovery. In the months that followed, her progress was slow but steady. She relearned how to connect her thoughts to her voice, eat, and eventually walk again.

Pam shared some remarkable stories about her experience from the other side, including some of her dreams and her ability to see what was going on all around her in the hospital. With the help of one of her friends, Deborah, Pam was able to document parts of her remarkable experience.

Over time, Pam regained her strength and was able to help plan Danielle's baby shower. The timing couldn't have been better. The birth of a child was the ultimate joy the family needed after nearly losing Pam. By the time the shower rolled around, Pam was walking on her own and had resumed some of her daily activities.

On the day of the baby shower, Pam looked beautiful in her pink top, white pedal pushers, and pink Croc-like, garden shoes. I told her I loved her shoes, and she said, "Thank you, but I have to change them before the others get here because my sister told me I couldn't wear them."

Being the comfort queen, I laughed and asked why not. I suggested she wear them until her sister arrived, and then she could change them. That's when she told me her sister wasn't coming, and I said, "Well then, she'll never know." Pam ended up wearing the pink clogs all day and shined in them!

Pam's grandson, Mark, was born in the summer of 2007. Pam and Dave were the proudest of grandparents. They were so happy and felt blessed. However, a few weeks later, Pam's leukemia returned with a vengeance, and she ended up back in the same ICU room where she had experienced that miracle just months before — the same machines, nurses, and doctors.

This time, we all knew it was Pam's time. She said she was just so grateful to have had the remission and extra time to be part of the planning, celebrating, and the birth of Mark. She was filled with love and resolve.

My feeling about Pam's miraculous remission is that it was a gift from the universe for the whole family — a temporary free pass for living a little longer so she could welcome her first grandchild. As mentioned in other chapters, everyone waits for that one thing. I believe Pam waited for Mark to be born, and the universe beautifully supported her.

Saying Goodbye

After a few days of being back on life support, the family honored Pam's final wishes and permitted the doctors to turn off all the machines. It was a devastatingly painful decision and such a brave thing for them to do.

I asked the family if I could stop by to say goodbye to my dear friend, and they all agreed. I arrived within minutes of the machines being turned off to find the three of them gathered around Pam — each writing messages of love and drawing pictures on her body with colored markers.

I moved through the room with gentleness and respect for their process and then leaned in to kiss Pam's forehead as my tears anointed her resting body. I thanked her for our friendship and expressed how much I loved her before saying goodbye. Witnessing her family's love surrounding her in those final moments was one of the most intimate experiences in my life.

Pam's Pink Shoes

After Pam's passing, her daughters asked if there was anything I wanted from her things. I said, "Yes, if you don't mind, I would like her pink shoes." I knew Pam would appreciate my request.

One of the other things I asked for was a picture of Pam in a full-length coat standing in the middle of a labyrinth. Dave had taken the photo on one of their beloved road trips. That picture still holds a prominent place in my home, where to this day, Pam and I continue our Wise Woman conversations whenever we want.

I proudly wore Pam's pink garden shoes, like Dorothy's ruby slippers, to her family's Celebration of Life gathering. I could feel Pam smiling down at me. I will always be grateful to my dear friend for freely sharing her humor, wisdom, spirit, and friendship.

CHAPTER 8

ANIMALS AS HEALERS AND TEACHERS

Our pets can be excellent teachers and healers, especially when it comes to end-of-life care and a soul's completion. The following two stories are about a stallion (and his human handler) and a desert tortoise. One is an example of an animal's ability to facilitate emotional healing for those suffering from a terminal illness. The other reflects an example of nature's cycle of life through the act of hibernation — a seasonal rest, replenishment, and preparation for spring rebirth. We can learn so much about death by witnessing nature's life cycles.

Most animals are sensitive and aligned with both the spirit and physical worlds. There is an energetic connection between animals and humans that allows us to communicate with each other through the silent network of thought and body language that can be healing for both. The title of "service animal" is well deserved for its generosity of spirit and ability to give unconditional love, emotional comfort, and a sense of safety. If you have ever spent time with an animal, you know exactly what I am talking about — it's a special type of bond.

"Horses remind us of who we truly are as they require our presence, evoke our joy, celebrate our authenticity, and return us to our innocence." ~ Kate Neligan

The Healing Power of Animals

A beautiful example of one animal's innate healing nature is a heartwarming story about a fifteen-year-old retired show-horse known by the medical team at Calais Hospital as "Doctor Peyo."[6] This beautiful stallion has an unusual gift of intuitively detecting an emotional or physical imbalance in humans, such as a tumor or cancer.

Peyo and his handler, Hassen Bouchakour, live in Northern France, where they spend a couple of days a week visiting hospitals and hospice centers helping terminally ill patients prepare for and integrate with the process of dying.

Hassen walks Peyo through the halls of the facilities where the stallion decides which patients (usually the sickest) he will visit by stopping at their door and lifting or stomping his foot. Hassen opens the door and leads Peyo into the room where he can assess his patient. The horse will then initiate a kiss, a stare, or a nuzzle in specific places on their body that almost always triggers an emotional response. This interaction appears to be an energetic soul release and healing that offers the patient and their family support and comfort. Sometimes, he will stand to watch over his patients for hours as they prepare to die.

Despite Doctor Peyo's large size, this empathetic animal moves through the halls with the grace of a Buddhist monk. At the time of the publication of this book, the duo assists approximately 20 patients each month, and scientists at the Calais Hospital are

---

6 The Guardian. (2022, October 19). *'Doctor Peyo': the horse comforting cancer patients in Calais — in pictures.* https://www.theguardian.com/society/gallery/2021/mar/12/doctor-peyo-the-horse-comforting-cancer-patients-in-calais-in-pictures

studying Peyo's healing ability. His presence and interactions at the facilities have been shown to reduce the stress and anxiety of everyone (patients, caregivers, family members) and, in some cases, the patient's need for medication.

Ms. Myrtle's Story

Ms. Myrtle is a California desert tortoise and my beloved pet. I met her when I was 19 while living in Nichols Canyon. She belonged to my neighbor, Bud Ekins, a legendary Hollywood stuntman and world-champion motorcycle racer. He rescued her during a race in the Mojave Desert, where the two of them went on to win.

When Bud died in 2007, I adopted Ms. Myrtle. Our first few years together were about getting to know each other's personalities and habits. To my surprise, she was very social, loved being massaged, and always enjoyed hanging out with my friends. Soon my neighbors and clients, along with their children, would stop by to visit Ms. Myrtle. They would come and sit in the garden with her — people love to watch her eat.

I was familiar with the healing abilities of service animals but never thought of a tortoise as a creature that would fall into that category. However, in watching people's body language when they were around her, I realized that Ms. Myrtle had a gift for healing peoples' emotional states. Some people were initially afraid of her, but after being in her presence for a while, their fear would dissipate. Watching and interacting with her brought them into the present moment — like a meditation — which appeared to have a calming effect on them and produce a greater sense of well-being.

Hibernation — A Lesson About Death and Rebirth

In addition to Ms. Myrtle's relaxing effect on people (and the neighborhood cats), she has also taught me a lot about the cycle of life. In the fall of our first year together, when she started preparing for hibernation, I thought something was wrong with her. She stopped eating and drinking and rarely came out. Her eyes glazed over, and she wasn't responding to my voice or our guests anymore. I thought I had failed as a tortoise mom and that she was sick, or worse, dying.

Fearing the latter, I called the tortoise society, where they reassured me that her behavior was quite normal as she prepared for hibernation. Her body and organs would slowly shut down over two months, eventually settling into a sleep state where she remained quiet and motionless until the spring when her spirit re-emerged into the same body — a rebirth of sorts.

Watching Ms. Myrtle's annual hibernation period, I saw how similar it was to a human's process of the cycle of life and a soul's release for future incarnations. The experience offered me a new sense of insight and acceptance around death.

Honoring Our Animal Friends

The following two stories are about two of my friend's relationships with their animals and how they processed their deaths and celebrated their lives — much like honoring our human loved ones. People who don't have animals may not understand or appreciate these stories, but for those of us who do, I hope Sandy and Kate's thoughts offer you some inspiration for acknowledging and celebrating your own pet's memory and life.

"Until one has loved an animal, a part of one's soul has not been awakened." ~ Anatole France

Sandy's Reflection of Oscar: The Handsome One

Oscar was a rescue dog who resembled Tramp from the Disney movie *Lady and the Tramp*. Whenever we took in another rescue, we'd enlist an animal communicator to help us integrate them into our household. Oscar would routinely start the session with the facilitator by bragging about his fur and then go on to say, "That's the new dog in our family, but I am the handsome one."

Oscar suffered from a degenerative leaky mitral heart valve as he got older. When he turned 16 and moved into his final days, our vet told us that it was time to emotionally prepare ourselves to let him go. If you have ever loved an animal, you know that sometimes we keep them alive because it is so hard to say goodbye. But after our conversation with the vet, we knew it was time.

Once we processed our feelings, we called the Hearts and Halos home pet euthanasia service to schedule a visit the following day to assist with Oscar's transition. Early the next morning, we prepared a burial space under the orange tree in our backyard. We carried Oscar outside and laid his little labored body on a blue blanket by the tree.

Next to Oscar, I placed red rose petals and orange pieces, along with his favorite stuffed toy, a bundle of sage, a love stone, a crystal, a seashell, and an essential oil mixture for animals (made by a friend) that we had been using to make him more comfortable.

A kind British woman from the pet service arrived a few minutes later through the side gate. She had never met Oscar before, but we knew right away she was the perfect gentle soul to usher our sweet boy home when she greeted him with, "Oh, my goodness, you are so handsome." That loving affirmation from a stranger was the last thing Oscar heard, and yes, indeed, he was the "handsome one."

She administered one shot, and he went to sleep … no pain or suffering, nothing but a smooth transition. We sat with his spirit, and I anointed his body with rose oil as we prayed and thanked him for his unconditional love, and the joy he brought us.

Later that day, I wrapped his body in a pair of my pajamas, and we lowered him into the earth with all of his altar offerings. Oscar now rests peacefully in the yard near his favorite orange tree, surrounded by what he loves.

I miss you so much, Buddy Love — always in our hearts. I am sure Bailey met you at the Rainbow Bridge, and you are romping and playing like the old days. Thank you for spending your life with us.

Kate and Lindsey: A Celebration of Life

Kate is a life and career coach who teaches her clients about confidence, teamwork, and overcoming fear through interacting with animals. Working with her horse Lindsey, Kate facilitated transformational change for her clients using experiential and intuitive processes similar to Peyo and Hassen's partnership.

In 2017, Kate noticed something wrong with Lindsey's rear left foot. The vet found a significant break in an untreatable spot. She was devastated and faced with a decision no one wants to make — what course of action to take.

While Kate viewed death as a blessing for the soul and the natural process of transitioning home, she was also confused about whether it was Lindsey's time. Wrestling with her sadness and indecision, she asked the universe and Lindsey herself for a clear sign to help her make this heartbreaking decision.

Shortly after, Lindsey's previous caretaker appeared serendipitously and offered her support. Kate knew at that moment what she needed to do and found the courage to stay with Lindsey and usher her through the entire process. Lying in the dirt by her side, Kate stroked her soft coat as her sweet friend's soul was released from her equine body.

Lindsey's Memorial

Lindsey's memorial took place at the base of a beautiful canyon in the hills of old Agoura, California, near a big oak tree. Kate created an altar in the middle of a large circle filled with memories of Lindsey, including a braided clipping of her tail. We later passed it around as a "talking stick" and shared our thoughts of gratitude for her life.

Each woman who attended brought something special to the circle — a message, a prayer, a token memory, or a new gift. Kate read a loving poem about one of the greatest lessons her friendship with Lindsey had given them both: the gift of being enough. One of their clients performed a healing sound bath with crystal bowls while we meditated. Kate shared how days before her passing, Lindsey had expressed her love of the crystal bowls by stomping her foot and dropping her nose into them to absorb the vibration from the sound waves.

Kate's Reflection

At the end of the service, a magnificent horse approached our circle with his human and greeted us, almost like Lindsey had sent us a thank-you gift. While my heart was both full and breaking at the same time, I was so grateful for the support of my friends and that my mother was in town to help me through it.

Having this life celebration for Lindsey was deeply healing for all of us. Many of us felt Lindsey's spirit running free in the mountains around us during the meditation.

For more information about Kate's healing work with humans and animals, visit kateneligan.com.

SALLY: MY NEIGHBOR
ACTIVIST & ANIMAL LOVER

Vignette Eight

♥

Sally was the first person I helped through transition outside of my family circle, and my first encounter with a visual manifestation of an animal spirit — Sally's beloved cat, Tio — when he came to greet her. I also learned that even after people are gone, their angelic souls can beautifully support us by keeping a promise they made while they were here — from the other side.

Sometimes you have a friend who knows what they want, but they need help fulfilling their wishes. My friend Sally was one of those people. I met Sally when my (then) husband and I bought the house next door to her in the San Fernando Valley. During escrow, it was mandatory to fumigate for termites, so I needed to find a creative, non-toxic way to get the job done.

The first time I saw Sally was when the service tech from the safe termite company arrived. As he pulled into our driveway, she poked her head out the front door, looking puzzled. After we introduced ourselves, Sally told me she was thrilled to meet me, as not many people knew about the electro-gun termite technology, and only a few were brave enough to try it. Sally had used the same company when she had moved in the previous year. We knew then we were kindred spirits and became trusted friends for the next 23 years.

Sally lived alone and was an activist for women's rights and seniors. Even though she leaned left politically, she worked on the

Governor's Task Force in supporting seniors' best interests under two Republican administrations from 1992-1999.

A few years after the 1994 Northridge earthquake, Sally was diagnosed with breast cancer. She chose surgery with a follow-up treatment of radiation and chemotherapy. Fortunately, one of her girlfriends could care for her until she regained her health.

Once Sally was back on her feet and in remission, she adopted a cat named Tio and a dog called Get-A-Long from the shelter. They brought her great joy and were her faithful companions, or as she referred to them, her "kids." She also started playing guitar and would practice for hours performing for the animals, Danielle, and me. She and my daughter became very close through the years, so much so that Sally was known to get stern with her like an auntie when necessary.

Get-A-Long passed away in 2007, and Tio had to be put to sleep later that same year. Both animals lived rich lives full of love under Sally's care. Once they were gone, she planted a beautiful rose bush outside her den door in their honor, which she watered religiously.

When Cancer Returns

Early one morning in June of 2008, Sally knocked on my door in tears. She asked me if I could take her to the hospital the following day for a procedure. She explained that she had been having trouble swallowing for a few months, but eating in the past few weeks had become impossible, and she was starving to death.

The following day, a multitude of tests revealed Sally had throat cancer. This particular cancer was very aggressive; she was already in an advanced stage and told there was no cure. Her doctor's only recommendation was to admit her to the hospital, where they could feed her through a tube and make her comfortable.

Sally told me she was tired of hospitals and doctors, and that wasn't how she wanted to spend her remaining time. I took her home and whipped up one of my favorite fruit smoothies, which filled her tummy and felt good on her throat.

When I checked on her the next morning, she was extremely depressed and confused. We ended up talking for hours. During that conversation, I asked her what she wanted to do. Her response was to complete her last days resting in the comfort of her own home. She didn't want to burden anyone or have anybody stay in her house.

Sally's brother and sister-in-law lived an hour away, but as close as she and her brother were, she still hadn't told him about her symptoms or diagnosis. Sometimes people with a fear of terminal illness believe if they don't acknowledge or talk about their symptoms, they'll magically go away. This tactic, however, only leads to a state of perpetual denial.

Making a Plan

When I asked Sally if she had a plan, she said her affairs were in order, but she wasn't sure how to fulfill her wish of staying home. After some contemplation, I came up with an idea and proposed that if I took care of her in this final phase, she would take care of me from the other side by bringing me wonderful new neighbors. She laughed. (I was grateful she could still laugh between her tears.) Having respectful, kind neighbors was very important to me. Sally had been a supportive and amazingly quiet neighbor over the years — a rarity.

Sally thought about it for a while and said, "Yes, I think I can do that for you."

I replied, "Great. Then we have a deal."

Sally and I quickly solidified our plan. She would call her brother and let him know about her cancer, and I would care for her as long as I could, making her protein shakes and broth and checking on her throughout the day. I would also be the liaison to her family, keeping them up-to-date throughout the process. Sally organized the rest of her paperwork within 24 hours, and her brother came up the following afternoon to meet with both of us to discuss all the details of her final wishes. We were all in agreement.

An Animal Spirit's Greeting

The following morning when I looked out my bedroom window, I was surprised to see a cat that looked exactly like Sally's Tio. He was sitting in the same spot he used to in my yard, staring at the back of her house just like when he was alive. My first thought was that Tio's spirit had come to greet Sally, but I had never seen the physical manifestation of a deceased soul before and questioned what I saw. I didn't think much about it until later when Sally told me she had seen Tio that morning. Then in a very matter-of-fact way, she stated that he had come to greet her, as animals do. I was so amazed that we had both seen him. After that sighting and greeting, I never saw that cat again.

At the beginning of the second week, Sally asked me to water her plants. I took care of the ones in the house but hadn't yet watered the mulberry bush that her brother had given her or the rose bush she had planted in memory of her beloved animals — both of which were in the backyard.

I took care of as many of her requests as possible in a timely manner while also keeping up with my own commitments. Sally's personal health needs and safety were my primary concerns, and I was fairly overwhelmed, so I never remembered to water her outdoor plants.

By the end of that week, Sally was deep into the transition process, and it was time to bring in hospice, a hospital bed, and a full-time nurse. Speaking became painful, so all verbal communication with her stopped; even writing down her thoughts or needs became too exhausting.

I continued to visit every few hours, even after hiring a full-time caregiver, to ensure she was comfortable. If Sally were awake when I came by, she would smile, mouth her request, or motion to let me know what she needed. Our time together was very special.

Everything was in place for Sally as we moved into the Fourth of July weekend. The timing coincided with my preparation to adopt a 50-year-old desert tortoise, Ms. Myrtle. (You met her earlier in this chapter.) Sally knew about the adoption, and we were both anxiously awaiting her arrival. At one point, I even thought she might be waiting to meet Myrtle before passing, so I continued to give her pick-up day updates and turtle yard-proofing progress reports.

Myrtle arrived on Friday, but Sally was still with us on Saturday, so I assumed that wasn't what she was waiting for to feel complete. This was in the early stages of my full understanding of how to clearly communicate with those in transition. To me, everything looked like it was in order, so Sally's one thing remained a mystery. When I went to sleep that night, I asked the universe for guidance in figuring out Sally's unfinished business.

The following morning, it came to me. I hadn't yet watered her important plants outside. So, after securing Myrtle's new environment, I went to Sally's and began watering all the plants. I watered trees and flowers that hadn't seen water in years other than the winter's rain. As I took care of each plant in the house, I would go into Sally's room and tell her which ones were complete. I knew she understood because she smiled each time.

I was down to the last two most important plants, her brother's mulberry bush and Tio and Get-A-Long's roses. The rose bush was right outside the room where Sally was resting, and I intentionally spoke to her through the screen door, "Sally, I'm watering your kids' plant. I'm giving it lots of love and water! Everything is taken care of now."

Once all the plants were well hydrated, I returned to Sally's room, where she was wrapped in her white sheets and now had a peaceful look on her face. I felt a sense of completeness knowing I had finished fulfilling all her requests. I gently stroked and kissed her forehead and told her one last time how grateful I was for our friendship. And I assured her I'd watch over the house and yard until the new owners arrived. I also reminded her about our deal regarding the new neighbors, and she gave me one last smile with her eyes still closed.

As I walked out of her house and back into my garden, I could hear my landline phone ringing. It had been no more than two minutes. When I heard the hospice worker's voice on the other end, I realized that Sally had taken her last breath, knowing everything was complete.

Honoring Sally

After calling Sally's brother, I returned to her house and gathered some mulberries with leaves attached, a rose, and a few sprigs of lavender, which I tied together in a bouquet and placed on her peacefully resting body.

While I was out in the yard gathering the flowers, I again heard the phone ringing at my house. When I got home, there was a message on my answering machine from my daughter — she wanted to tell me about a strange experience she had just had. When I called Danielle back, she was crying and said she dreamt that Sally had come to say goodbye. She whispered, "Thank you for our friendship," and told Danielle she wanted her to enjoy her guitar. It was a very powerful experience for my daughter, and I was amazed by their connection in that moment of release.

Sally's brother and sister-in-law arrived an hour later, and they embraced the sacredness of spending time with Sally for a few more hours before letting her physical body go.

Sally's Promise

Within five months, Sally fulfilled her promise to me by bringing a family of four that would honor her memory and be lovely new neighbors. It also turned out that the family and I had several mutual friends. Fifteen years later, her mulberry bush continues to flourish with tasty berries, and the rose bush is watered regularly.

CHAPTER 9

LOSS & GRIEF

"Honoring our grieving process and that of others allows us to be present with our hearts. It opens a space for reflection that might have otherwise been closed." ~ Kathy Arnos

Sitting With the Feelings — The Tears That Heal Us

Grief is a natural response that arises from a loss or circumstances that are emotionally painful and out of our control. Interestingly, on some level, we spend a good portion of our lives in this uncomfortable emotional state. The depth of it will vary based on the situation — the loss of a family member, friend, an animal, a body part; a disappointment, divorce, miscarriage, a child going off to college, leaving one job for another, some form of betrayal, a lifestyle change, or a geographic move. The list is endless.

Grief is sneaky; at times, even unrecognizable, and we don't even know we are in the thick of it. The Covid pandemic of 2020 was unlike anything my generation or younger had ever experienced. It was an unprecedented example of loss, including our freedom, where we all grieved together. As I mourned with the rest of the world, I also felt empathetic grief for those around me — those who had lost loved ones and others struggling to feed their families or were evicted from their homes.

I felt disappointed with the deficiencies in the medical and economic systems that were not equipped to meet the crisis. I also witnessed a sense of desperation in people I had never seen before — locally and worldwide. The pandemic impacted everyone. Trying to make sense of the changing facts and protocols and the uncertainty and chaos surrounding it was confusing. And unfortunately, some friendships imploded over differing responses to and beliefs about the crisis.

Recognizing that moment as a true form of grief amongst the fear was difficult because it was a different kind of loss. Once I understood that what I was feeling was depression associated with grief, I began talking to others about it and found they were experiencing similar feelings. Those conversations were helpful and small pods of like-minded people emerged to support each other through those challenging times. Similar to a support group for the bereaved.

As I mentioned earlier, I never had that kind of emotional support as a child. No one asked me how I was feeling or dared to talk to me about my loss. There were only whispers behind my back and silence in my presence.

I hid my sadness and would wait until everyone was in bed at night before crying myself to sleep. I was ashamed of my feelings, lived with constant anxiety and depression, and routinely had bad dreams — all of which were normal responses to the trauma of losing a parent. It was a surreal period that could have had a much healthier outcome if someone had talked to me and given me the support needed to understand my feelings and help me start processing my grief.

Today, I understand how important it is to take time to mourn our losses and direct others who need help processing their feelings to appropriate resources. Grief is a complex and multifaceted emotion that can impact our mind, body, and spirit and is normal and essential to our healing process. Everyone will do it differently. Elisabeth Kubler-Ross wrote extensively about grief and its five prominent stages — denial, anger, bargaining, depression, and acceptance — which I have found can be applied to all experiences of loss.

While there is great emphasis on these five stages, Kübler-Ross originally introduced them as a loose framework to support those who were dying so they could understand how to process their feelings and begin a healthy, honest conversation with those around them.

However, death and grieving expert David Kessler, who co-authored two books with Kübler-Ross, reminds us not to reduce our grief to these stages alone - they simply describe general patterns. Other essential stages include anticipatory (anxiety) and yearning (longing and emptiness) grief.

Even though Kessler had been working with dying and grieving families for many decades, in 2016, he experienced and learned about an even deeper level of loss when one of his sons died suddenly — a pain he had never known. That's when he wrote *Finding Meaning: The Sixth Stage of Grief* as part of his healing process.

Besides the more obvious signs of grief, such as uncontrollable tears and overwhelming sadness, behavior changes to watch for include an overall sense of malaise — a person not wanting to get out of bed, isolating, overwhelmed by being around people, anxiety or panic attacks, feelings of insecurity, avoiding phone calls, loss of appetite, lack of interest in friends, work or hobbies and mood swings. These are just a few of the more common symptoms.

Also, these stages aren't necessarily specific to time frames or sequences. Everyone's journey is unique. Each time I cared for someone in transition, I found that I grieved differently. Sometimes it began with the diagnosis; other times, it was more pronounced towards the end or after they were gone.

For those who experience loss abruptly through a tragic accident, suicide, or an unexpected death from natural causes, the grieving process is very different because they also deal with the added emotional shock and trauma of the situation. There is no closure, kiss goodbye, or last conversation — their loved ones simply disappear into the abyss. In the case of suicide, there are usually many unanswered questions, and we will never fully understand their pain. Also, the stigma around death by suicide is tremendous, so for those left behind, feelings of shame, guilt, regret, or what-ifs can be consuming.

These types of death are infinitely more complicated and require special care to assist with recovery and healing. There are several insightful books specific to grief related to different types of sudden loss, from natural causes, trauma, or suicide, some of which are listed in the Resources at the end of the book.

"Grief, I've learned, is really just love. It's all the love you want to give, but cannot. All that unspent love gathers up in the corners of your eyes, the lump in your throat, and in that hollow part of your chest. Grief is just love with no place to go."
~ Jamie Anderson

Processing The Feelings

I encourage people to talk about their feelings, whether with a friend, a support group, a grief community, or a religious or spiritual leader or group — just find someone. These deep feelings are not something that can be ignored or processed alone.

Healing takes time (months or years), on your time and no one else's. Acknowledge the loss and be with the feelings as they arrive — give it all the space it needs. Eventually, a new chapter will begin — as reflected in the 2020 pandemic. Amidst the sadness and hardship, there were also positive things that came about due to the loss people experienced.

Business and school closures and stay-at-home orders gave people more quality time for connection and reflection. Many reevaluated their priorities, lives, careers, and relationships while developing more meaningful bonds with their friends and loved ones.

People parked their cars and got out in nature (riding their bikes, walking, camping, etc.), and the environment and relationships began to heal. The long-overdue reality check regarding racial inequality was thrust into the forefront as people came together to support each other and rise against the injustices many have faced for so long. Beautiful acts of kindness popped up amongst all age groups across the world.

How we humans processed grief around this unprecedented event shared similarities with what happens when a loved one dies. It was a time of transformation — from despair to courage. I took a personal inventory, sold my house, moved cross country, and bought a new house in three months. It was about letting go of everything I knew and moving forward into the unknown — the death of the old into a rebirth of the new. It was one of the best things I could have done for myself.

The bottom line is if you or someone you know has recently gone through a loss and may be in trouble (displaying any of the aforementioned symptoms), please acknowledge the feelings, take action, and get help.

Below are some tools and resources to help guide you through the process.

Exercises & Resources for Healing

Daily routines are essential to the healing journey. Do at least one thing each day: shower, get dressed, make your bed, or have a meal. However small, it will be healing on some level. Other suggestions include:

- Join a grief group
- Journal your feelings
- Write a letter to your loved one
- Get out in nature — it brings you closer to heaven
- Exercise
- Meditate (can be solo or you can use guided meditations and visualizations about grief)
- Paint, draw, or connect to some form of expression of your feelings
- Laugh — laughter produces the release of positive chemicals in the brain and relaxes the central nervous system
- Sleep as much as you need to, as it is restorative and also helps you process unconscious feelings
- Embrace rituals, like lighting candles or creating an altar

- Honor your memories: find a token you can carry with you or have in your space, and hang up photos or quotes that support your feeling connected to your loved one
- Listen to music and/or dance (gentle movement) to release emotional blockages
- Schedule grieving time to let loose with your feelings in a safe environment
- Try the Emotional Freedom Technique (EFT) or "tapping" (learn more in the Resources.)
- Explore homeopathic remedies and flower essences for grief

Doing anything on this list will help move you forward and begin to heal your heavy heart and fractured spirit. There are more resources to help support you in the Grieving section of the Resources.

DAMION: LESSONS OF FORGIVENESS

Vignette Nine

♥

"I find myself choosing to just sit in God's lap and let Him hold me close for a while." ~ Author Unknown

Working with Damion, his mother, and his sister allowed me to learn about facilitating acts of forgiveness within a family dynamic for people I love deeply. I was able to check in with him and relay his wishes through direct conversations between them all. They, in turn, could use that information and connect with their intuition to be advocates for his best care. Being part of their process was such an honor and showed me that everyone deserves to be walked home with dignity and loving support no matter what challenges they have faced in life. The three of them were able to do that with forgiveness in their hearts and a true sense of completion. Damion died knowing how much he was loved.

Damion, my good friend Kathleen's son, was in his early 40s and had struggled with addiction since adolescence. Over the years, Damion's substance abuse landed him on the streets, where he spent a lot of time at a local church. There he met Lindah, a woman who ran its homeless rehabilitation program, with whom he developed a strong bond. Lindah became a great advocate for him, as she did for many of the others who would seek her help. Everyone called her Mama Lindah.

Damion had been experiencing headaches for a while, and at Mama Lindah's advice, he finally sought proper medical attention. The tests revealed he was suffering from MRSA bacteria in his brain and encephalitis, and he was immediately admitted to the hospital. He phoned his sister Dawnielle. When she asked how he was feeling, he responded, "I can't do this anymore. I am really tired. I am done, and Avi is here with me."

Dawnielle understood his lifelong fatigue yet thought his last statement was strange. Avi was their deceased grandfather, who had died years ago in that same hospital. Neither of them had spoken about him in years.

His mother and sister promptly booked flights from Northern California to be with him. Unfortunately, by the time they arrived, the doctors had already performed what they considered emergency brain surgery.

Thankfully, Damion was conscious and somewhat communicative when they arrived. He was able to squeeze their fingers to answer yes and no questions, and he used sign language to let them know he wanted one of his favorite pleasures — candy. His responsiveness gave the family hope for his recovery.

After spending the day with her brother and seeing his progress, Dawnielle decided to return home to care for her kids and left the following day. Kathleen stayed with Damion to continue monitoring his condition. Unfortunately, his abilities quickly began to deteriorate. Despite the doctor's and nurses' efforts to continue his rehabilitation therapy, he could no longer communicate or participate. As Kathleen's hope faded, she decided to call upon two of our friends for advice, Clifton and Lynne — both holistic practitioners.

Further Assistance Needed

I received a text from Clifton on Saturday morning asking if I had spoken to Kathleen lately. When I said I hadn't, he shared what little information he had about the situation but said things weren't looking good for Damion. He knew I had experience in this area and felt I might be better able to assist them.

When looking for guidance in assessing a situation, I listen for subtle details in people's stories. I called Kathleen for more information about his condition, requesting any pictures or videos she had taken of him.

Within minutes of our conversation, Kathleen told me how, ironically, she had just run into the woman who cared for her mother-in-law during her last phase at the same hospital. Kathleen hadn't seen this woman since her passing and thought it was an odd coincidence that she would be visiting a friend at that moment. I saw this as a clear signal from the universe about Damion's transitional status.

Kathleen also sent me a video of Damion. Shortly after reviewing it, I began receiving messages from him. I heard the words, "I am really tired. I don't want to do this anymore. I am done."

I had no idea he had already verbalized these same sentiments to Dawnielle.

I suggested Kathleen return to the hospital to discuss his situation and prognosis again with his doctor. Given all of the clues: the chance encounters, his words, seeing his grandfather, the messages I was receiving, and the video, it was no surprise that he was no longer responding to treatment. I suggested that perhaps Damion was more inclined towards hospice care than rehabilitation.

Kathleen told me she felt the same way but didn't know what to do about it. When medical professionals tell you one thing, and you feel differently —perhaps even guilty for your opposing thoughts — it can be confusing. It's essential to have someone to talk to who can help you think through the situation.

Kathleen needed someone to give her permission and a little courage to speak her truth to the doctors, and I was able to offer her that help. I received a text from her an hour later letting me know that the doctors had agreed and would be taking Damion off life support and moving him into hospice care later that night. They assured her they would make him comfortable.

Kathleen then asked if I would call Dawnielle and talk to her. Often, when a family faces these difficult decisions, it is hard to know what to do. Dawnielle was very upset and confused. She couldn't decide whether or not to arrange for childcare again and fly back down. I told her I understood her dilemma but suggested her mother needed her support. No one should go through something like this alone, and I didn't want her to regret not being part of her brother's transition (even if he passed before she got there).

Later that night, Kathleen texted me to let me know that after a long day of paperwork and challenging logistics, Damion had finally settled into his hospice room. He was resting comfortably, and she was going home for the night.

Dawnielle arrived the following morning, and she and her mother did what they could to ensure Damion would be comfortable throughout his process. After speaking with the three of them, I realized there might still be some unresolved feelings from the past between them that needed to be healed.

Having spent time with homeless people, especially those with addiction, I know that many feel a great deal of shame and a sense of being a burden to their families. I knew how much both of these women loved Damion and thought it was important for him to understand that they accepted and loved him for who he was despite their frustration with his disease.

I offered them suggestions for a dialog to help shift any leftover negative energy patterns and allow space to move forward. I suggested they tell Damion exactly what would be happening on their end over the next 24 hours and that they had taken care of everything for him to experience a smooth transition. They both had commitments in their own lives and would be leaving the following day, so the rest was entirely up to him, whether he wanted to go while they were still there or after they had gone. Either way would be perfectly fine. I encouraged them to tell him that he controlled this final decision. It was his choice.

Let the Music Play On

Even though neither Dawnielle nor Kathleen had ever experienced this type of telepathic communication, they willingly embraced the opportunity by asking me questions via phone or text. Damion had quite a sense of humor, especially when they texted me to ask if there was something they could read to him. He quickly responded, "Oh please, don't let them read to me. I want music!"

I asked what his favorite band was, and Kathleen streamed it on her phone and played it throughout the afternoon. Damion was so happy, as were all of us at our respective locations. The love we all felt that day was so beautiful and heartwarming.

Once everything appeared to be in order, I asked Damion if there was anything else he was waiting for to feel complete. He said, "I am still waiting for her." I kept asking him who she was, but he just kept repeating, "Her."

I called Kathleen and told her he was waiting for a woman, but he wasn't specific. I asked if she could think of anyone he might need to complete with or want to see. After the call, Kathleen didn't respond for almost a full day, but finally, I received a text from her with a picture of a woman lying next to Damion. In my mind, I heard him say, "She's here, thank you."

I later realized that in her silence, Kathleen was holding space for her son, and it enabled her to tap into Damion's desire to see his ex-wife Mia before leaving his physical body. She was one of the good things in his life that had fallen apart because of his addictions and the behavior that goes with them.

Kathleen called Mia, and she immediately came to his bedside to say goodbye. They needed to forgive each other for things that had happened in their relationship over the years. After that healing and forgiveness took place between them, Damion was complete.

Once Kathleen saw he was content, she said her final goodbyes to her beloved son and headed to the airport to catch her flight. As she left, she felt a deep sense of gratitude for this time with Damion and their completion and held a prayer for his smooth transition. Shortly after returning home, Kathleen received a call from the hospital letting her know that Damion had passed and was at peace.

A Celebration of Damion's Life

Damion's friends and family honored him on World Mental Health Day at Mama Lindah's Lighthouse Church. Friends from different stages of his life were there with live music courtesy of various musicians who played some of Damion's favorite songs.

One homeless woman shared how Damion had always made her feel loved. One night when she was sitting outside a 99 Cents Store feeling cold, alone, and hopeless, Damion came along with his guitar and sang to her until the sun came up. She felt like she wouldn't have made it through that night had he not been there for her. Her story reminded me of something Maya Angelou once said about how people will never forget how you made them feel. I believe Damion's actions offered this homeless woman a sense of importance and of being seen and heard.

Later that evening, while talking with some family members, I felt Damion's presence all around me and sought out the woman he had sung to. I told her how much I enjoyed her story and felt sure Damion would always watch over her, his arms around her like a guardian angel. She cried and gave me a long, warm hug. She was thrilled with that thought!

CHAPTER 10

MESSAGES FROM BEYOND:
GUIDANCE, GIFTS & VISITATIONS

In this section, I ask that you open your minds and hearts to the realm of unknown possibility — the mystery and the unexplainable. Because you're reading this book, chances are you are ready to take the journey with me from the intellectual mind into the spiritual realm of possibility.

The following personal stories will allow you to explore the idea of being open to receiving messages from beyond. My goal is not to convince you of anything but rather to share some of my own experiences and those of others, which I wholeheartedly believe to be interactions with loved ones on the other side. It's up to you to decide whether or not they are a coincidence or a message from beyond.

Humans communicate in many tangible ways — through technology, body, sign, and written language, verbally, etc. There is also the energetic or biochemical network of transmission throughout the animal kingdom and nature — plants and trees — the quantum realm. More of these invisible communication systems are being discovered and studied by the scientific community all the time. Interacting with the spirit world via unseen channels is simply part of this remarkable web of conversation.

As you will see reflected in the stories, once someone we love is gone, they may interact with us in creative ways, using scents, music, lights, technology, humor, or the words of someone else — the list is endless — and usually happens when we least expect it.

The signs can be bold and recognizable or very subtle. Some messages will be a form of guidance, while others simply let us know that their spirits are still very much with us.

Today, I have friends who frequently call with great excitement to share their stories of interaction, while the non-believers politely tolerate my strangeness. However, I have found that after speaking with someone wavering in their beliefs on the subject, I will often receive a call or email shortly after telling me about something that happened to them. New pathways are formed by having this awareness, providing a gentle opening to view the afterlife in ways they could never have imagined.

I feel blessed to have this rare gift and connection with the spirit world. But not everyone will experience these interactions consciously or tangibly as I do — and that's okay. You are not being left out of the cosmic gift pool. I encourage you to embrace the idea that your loved one's spirit is always engaged in this dimensional activity, whether you realize it or not. They love you and are still there silently supporting your highest good.

Spirit Sightings

The mother of one of my good friends from high school was a medium, and there was never a shortage of playful spirit activity at her house. My friend was the eldest of six kids, so there were always chores to be done. Since I was there often, mine was usually vacuuming. The only problem was that whenever I would approach a particular sitting area in her mother's bedroom, the vacuum would shut off.

One day I had this vision of a jovial man's spirit lounging on the loveseat with a cocktail in his hand. When I told my friend that the vacuum kept turning off, she laughed and said, "Oh, that's where Caesar hangs out. He has a great sense of humor, so just clean around him." My friend went on to describe him exactly as I had seen him.

"The silence of the night brings great opportunities of connection to the spirit realm simply because the distractions of the day are sleeping." ~ Kathy Arnos

Rose: *Guidance From My Stepmother*

The two strongest communications I received from my stepmother Rose came at different times. The first was shortly after she passed when my accountant recommended that I seek the advice of a financial adviser for my future planning. I wasn't totally on board with the idea, but I respected my accountant and agreed to meet the man.

Finances: His office was on the eighth floor of a high-rise building with a view of the valley. It was a windy day, and I could see big tree branches flying through the air in the distance. Just as I was getting ready to sign the proposed agreement, a small sparrow-like bird with a yellow breast landed outside on a one-inch window ledge right next to me and began frantically pecking at the window and chirping. It was as if it were yelling at me.

In the past, I had received several messages from different types of birds — usually representing good fortune; notably one on my wedding day and another on the day my daughter was born. This bird reminded me of my stepmother, and I felt it was trying to warn me about something. The relentless bird stayed on that ledge despite the howling winds, staring directly at me, screeching and pecking. I didn't heed its warning, and I signed the contract anyway, which later proved to be an unnecessary, costly mistake.

Approval: The second message came through during the same year and was very clear. I had been dating a lovely man (Dave) that both my parents knew, but he and I had never been romantically involved while they were alive. One night after dinner, I thought, *I wonder what my parents would think about our dating.* A few hours later, while we were watching television, we both heard a strange noise in the other room, like a metal object hitting something hard.

Walking down the long hallway to investigate the sound, I stepped on something hard that hurt my foot. When I turned on the light, I saw my stepmother's wedding ring in the middle of the floor. I had left it in the bathroom in the window box, which was around the corner and another eight feet away — a notably odd occurrence.

The dimensional beings, which I often referred to as the "Spirit Walkers," had always been very active in my house. However, I felt this was a very specific communication from my stepmother's spirit, giving her approval of this relationship.

Paula's Gifts in Paradise

Two days after Paula's passing, I boarded a plane to Hawaii. I was seated next to a little girl and her mother, and throughout the flight, their interactions reminded me of my relationship with my stepsister. Paula would often mistakenly call me "mommy." Toward the end of the flight, when the little girl introduced herself to me, I was surprised to learn she had the same last name as my sister, and I felt her presence right there with me.

Paula's spirit, playful energy, and many gifts entertained all of us the entire time we were in Hawaii. I felt they were a beautiful affirmation of her gratitude; thankfully, I was present enough to recognize them!

When we checked into our hotel, I was given a suite-sized room with the best view of the mountains and the ocean. It had an outdoor patio that overlooked a bird sanctuary, and I received a surprise room credit every day because I had opted out of daily cleaning services. I enjoyed several free meals with the credit.

My sister had a great sense of humor ... on the first day, my phone rang, and the caller ID said it was from Paula. I almost fainted! For a split second, I slipped into a time warp and thought maybe the hospital made a mistake, and she was still alive. Of course, that was not the case. When I answered it, my daughter's voice was on the other end. I had forgotten that I had sent her my sister's phone to use until her new one arrived.

The following day we took a day trip to Lanai, where our six-hour adventure turned into nine hours of pure magic. Our tour guide, Captain Kate, said she had never experienced this type of ocean activity in all her years of running tours on the Island. We were mesmerized by the extreme playfulness of the dolphins and a pod of whales (a male escort, a female, and a calf). I also scored the best seat on the boat at the helm sitting next to Captain Kate and her family, who were visiting from the mainland. We had an unrestricted view the whole trip back.

Each morning, I took long walks on the beach, where I was able to reflect and process my feelings about Paula's passing. There was rarely anyone out at dawn, but on New Year's morning, I met a couple at Black Rock Point that was also taking in the stillness of nature's beauty. The three of us stood knee-deep in the ocean as her husband videotaped the dawn.

Suddenly the woman pointed out a baby sea turtle swimming toward me. I stood very still, and it began swimming circles around me. As the currents of the waves pushed me in different directions, the little turtle continued to keep its rhythm following me.

A few minutes later, a bigger turtle, presumably the mother, appeared and began doing the same, following my every move, always keeping a couple of feet away. Eventually, I started back towards the hotel, slowly moving in the water. The turtles continued to follow me more than halfway home before disappearing out to sea.

When I got back to the hotel, two friends invited me to join them for breakfast and a few hours of snorkeling at my favorite cove. I wasn't so keen on eating at another crowded restaurant with long waiting times, but I wanted to visit the cove and spend time with my friends.

Our waitress was a lot of fun, and when I shared our frustration with finding a dinner reservation at a restaurant that served healthier food, she quickly asked how many were in our party and what time we would like to go. Her fiancé was the head chef at one of the finest restaurants on the island, and she said she would see what she could arrange for us. When she brought our check, she told us we were all set for dinner and gave us the address.

When we arrived, we were shown to a private cabana overlooking the beach, where we enjoyed a six-course meal of the most exquisitely prepared food I have ever tasted on the Island. (As a travel writer back in the nineties, I had written about some of the spa resorts in Hawaii.)

At the end of the night, a line of chefs emerged from the kitchen, each with a different dessert for us to try. It was incredible, and when they brought the bill, we discovered they hadn't charged us for any of the desserts, only the meal — the desserts were a gift.

Paula's last gift on the trip came when I boarded the plane home and was seated in a window seat. My preference for long flights has always been an aisle seat. A father and son sat down next to me, and I could see the little boy was very energetic and knew the flight wouldn't be relaxing.

I closed my eyes and thought, *I wish I were in a different seat.* A few minutes passed before the father asked if I would be open to changing places with his wife, who was also on the plane. I agreed, and it turned out that her seat was not only an aisle seat but it was right next to my friends. None of them could believe my luck. I laughed and thanked Paula for taking care of the situation for me, as well as delivering all of her wonderful surprises over the ten days!

Paula's Cane, Gabriel

When I was writing Paula's story, I got a message from her, reminding me that I hadn't yet included anything about her relationship with her walking cane. This was important to her because, in the end, it became her best friend, but neither of us could remember its name. I told Paula if she wanted his name to be included in the book, she'd have to remember it and let me know.

The following day when I was grocery shopping, I noticed a mother and daughter checking out in front of me who reminded me of my shopping experiences with Paula when she was alive. The daughter became impatient with her mother as she fumbled to put her money card away, then rushed out of the store — just like I used to do. The mother had rested her cane on the counter ledge and had forgotten it, just like Paula often did when we were out.

When I reached for the cane to give it back to the mother, I felt a bolt of energy move through my hand and up my arm as the words, "Gabriel, the cane's name is Gabriel!" flew out of my mouth. The cashier and mother thought I was crazy, but I didn't care and enthusiastically kept repeating, "The cane's name is Gabriel!" with great joy. Paula remembered it and beautifully orchestrated the perfect situation to give me the information. Praise Gabriel!

Moving With the Spirits

One night in mid-September 2021, a voice woke me up from a deep sleep saying it was time to sell my house and move to the Midwest. I laughed and said out loud, " I think you have the wrong person."

Suddenly, I felt my father's energy with me in the room, and his voice was very clear. *It's time for you to move, NOW.* Once I realized this was a serious instruction, I called my daughter the following day and told her of my experience and spontaneous, unexpected decision — she laughed and thought I was joking.

To everyone's shock and disbelief, my house was on the market within the week. After hearing my father's voice, I slipped into another zone, where I could let the universe's divine energy of flow move through me with faith to help me release my 34 years of attachment to my home and property that had served me well … including the labyrinth. It was the ultimate exercise of letting go and surrendering.

Within a few weeks, I was ready to accommodate a four-day-long open house. Each day, I would water the yard and labyrinth area before leaving. I used this time in open-house exile for meditation and to communicate with my father, asking him and what I called "The Committee" (God, Goddess, Spirit) for guidance and support with all the big decisions I would be making.

On the fourth day, I noticed a beautiful clear crystal-type stone with a variegated rainbow running through it next to the Goddess. I hadn't seen it before and knew it held a special message, but wasn't sure what it meant. I held it while I watered, and returned it to its original spot next to the statue of Grace before leaving the circle. I knew more would be revealed.

Out of the many offers I received the next day, there were three families for consideration. Two of the offers came with a beautiful letter of persuasion. We asked for a counteroffer to see what the next steps would be — the two with the letters went higher. The third family could not go higher but included a note this time. The man expressed his family's experience in visiting my home as follows: "When we first walked into your home, my wife had tears in her eyes. We have been looking for almost a year, and this is the first time we have fallen in love.

I am a Taoist, and Feng Shui is vital for us. Your home is beaming with good Feng Shui. We want a home to grow old in. We envision our daughter having her friends over and playing in the beautiful labyrinth in the backyard.

The three of us don't have relatives in Los Angeles, and our chosen family is within walking distance of the home. When our seven-year-old daughter, Gia, saw the house, she loved it. She even left a fairy stone in the hands of the lady sculpture in the backyard. We love everything about this home and would keep everything intact. We would be honored to live in your home and hope you choose us."

The list of similarities between our families was long — both men were of Greek origin, and collectively we all had similar professions. Also, my husband and I were not the highest bidders when we bought, and it was our first home. It was time to pay it forward. I later learned that Gia had made a wish on that fairy stone that my house would be their new home.

If you've read the vignette about my father, you already know about our strong connection to the labyrinth, so I knew Dad had a hand in orchestrating this divine alignment. I believe he (and "The Committee") had a great time organizing the cosmic energy for myself and this perfect family — a family who would fully appreciate the space.

Dave's Surprises

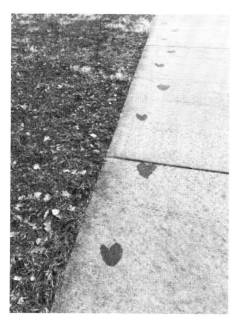

My dear friend and soulmate Dave, often surprises me with funny little gifts. Since his death, it seems like we have been in communication daily. I'm unsure if it's because he is one of the more recent departures or because of our deep soul connection — maybe both — whatever the reason, I love it.

Soothing my Grief: Shortly after Dave's passing, I was walking along a path in nature with a friend expressing how much I missed him. We had walked one way for about 45 minutes before turning around and returning the way we came. I was explaining the different ways one can receive messages from a deceased loved one when suddenly I felt a strong sense of Dave's presence. I paused, and when I looked down a trail of hearts was lining the pathway as far as we could see. I felt it was a beautiful affirmation of the process and a message of love from Dave that helped soothe my grieving heart.

Comfort: One of the last things Dave bought for his new house (and comfort) was a La-Z-Boy Recliner. One night shortly after his passing, I was sitting in the living room and thought, *I wish my furniture were more comfortable.*

A few days later, while looking for a new rug, I ended up at a furniture store in an aisle lined with recliners. It turned out my favorite one was also the La-Z-Boy brand. I had never sat in one and was surprised at how comfortable it was. I searched through the selection and couldn't find one that met my needs — the right color, material, and affordable — so I decided to let go of the thought that there was a recliner in my future.

One of the ladies I was with suggested that before we go, we should check out the clearance room, so off we went. As we approached the entrance, I saw a beautiful La-Z-Boy swivel recliner that was perfect in every way for only $299. When I sat in it, I heard Dave say, "Here you go — made to order!" I have found that since Dave's passing, I'll have a thought or telepathic conversation with the spirit world, and in a relatively short amount of time, I'll receive some type of response.

Legal Stuff: One day I found myself in a situation where I needed a specific legal document related to an arrangement I had with Dave, which was going to take a month to get. I needed it immediately and was feeling very stressed about it. The following morning during my meditation, I asked for the universe and spirits to support me in finding a creative solution. After lunch, I received a call from the woman who had requested the document. She said, "I am not sure how this happened, but we don't need the documentation anymore." And just like that, it was mysteriously resolved.

Humor: Dave always had a great sense of humor, and it seems to have carried over into the spirit realm. One night, there was a violent storm: the wind was howling, and there was an electrifying display of light in the night sky as Mother Nature's power shook the windows. I was dutifully standing in the kitchen watching the news to track potential tornados heading in my direction while deciding if I needed to move downstairs into the basement for shelter (aka

"Dave's Wing," which was filled with his favorite mission-style furnishings).

Suddenly, I saw a light come on from around the corner in the stairwell leading into the basement. At first, I was startled by it, but then I became curious. Motion activated, the sensor light at the top of the stairwell came on, but no one else was in the house. The next descending light came on within seconds as if someone were walking down the stairs. A couple of minutes passed, and the lights went off only to be reactivated, this time moving in the reverse as if someone were coming up the stairs. I burst into laughter, knowing this was Dave's shenanigans. It was as if he were saying, "Are you coming or not?" I chuckled and followed Dave's lead into the basement to safety.

A Transcript Message: After Dave's passing, I regularly listened to the only voicemail I had saved. Hearing his voice always brings me comfort. He had left it one month before he died. It was a rather silly message, and for some reason, he hadn't said "I love you" at the end of the call — something he usually did. I was envious that my daughter had several saved messages from him telling her he loved her.

A year later while listening to the message again, I noticed its transcript on my phone, which I had never seen before. To my surprise, it differed from his voice message, and the emotion "I love you" was right there all along.

Transcript: "Hi Kathy, it's Dave — call his phone — *I love you* — so well, it's Friday — (I'm) in the ground, oh gosh, call me — earlier time, eight o'clock — OK, I'll talk to you later."

Voice message: "Hi Kathy, it's Dave calling from my living room. It's Friday around, oh gosh, it's early your time, around eight o'clock, woof ... OK, I'll talk to you later." (Dave died around eight o'clock in the morning.)

The following stories come from friends who, like me, have enjoyed interactions with loved ones after they've dropped their physical bodies.

Laura: A Blanket of Sand Dollars

My dear friend, Laura, wasn't super close with her father, but the one place she would always find happy moments with him was sailing on the ocean, where he taught her how to navigate his sailboat. They lived in different states, yet once or twice a year, they always spent a few days reconnecting at sea.

During the summer of 1995, Laura found herself at an emotional crossroads and wanted to escape from her adult responsibilities. She needed some time to get quiet, think, and regroup. Her daughter was out of town, so she decided to take a few days off from work and drive up the coast.

In California, the beaches are always crowded in the summer, so Laura had to drive past Santa Cruz to find a secluded spot for the night. She waited for everyone to leave the beach before setting up her sleeping bag between two tall dunes and enjoying a little dinner. The night air was crisp, and the sky was clear and full of vibrant stars. It was exactly what she needed to get grounded and replenish her spirit.

The following day, Laura woke up at dawn and walked down to the water's edge, where she was greeted by one of the most magical sights she had ever seen. There before her was a magnificent blanket of sand dollars across the entire shoreline. The waves gently moved the delicate sea biscuits closest to the water around as they flowed in and out with the tides.

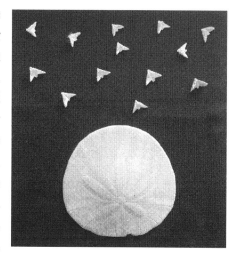

Laura felt like it was a message from the universe letting her know everything she had been stressing about would be okay. She was in awe and collected several as a memento of her experience. In the process, one of the treasures cracked open, and an array of little white birds emerged — a cherished moment of surprise and a beautiful display of nature's perfection.

When Laura returned home that evening, there was a message from a family member informing her that her father had suffered a heart attack and died that morning while he was sailing. When she realized that his death must have happened around the same time as her morning discovery, she felt that the star-designed creatures and emerging white birds were a parting gift from her father. Someone dying suddenly is always shocking, but she was so grateful that he went quickly doing something he loved — sailing on the ocean.

Kay: A Mother's Visitations

My friend Kay was visiting her mother a few months after her father, Ted, died when she unexpectedly began describing an unusual experience. Her mom had been lying in bed, facing away from the doorway, towards the wall, when she felt a presence. She stayed very still, saying she hadn't been frightened because she sensed Ted's spirit had entered the room.

Kay's mother felt a shift of weight as if Ted were getting into bed and lying next to her. Then she felt something drape across her waist like an arm embracing her, and she told him, "Ted, it's okay for you to go without me; you'll be okay. It's your time, not mine." After a moment, she felt something shift off her waist, the weight lifted from the bed, and Ted was gone.

This type of unexplainable phenomenon had never happened before, so Kay knew her mom's experience was very real. Kay also felt strongly her father needed her mother's reassurance and permission to feel complete before fully letting go.

Kay's mother lived another 28 years after Ted's passing. As Kay got older, she prayed that someday her mom would find someone who would love her for who she was and be good to her for the rest of her life.

Years later, Kay's mom moved to an assisted living facility, where she met a kind and loving man named Hal. Kay learned about Hal on Valentine's Day when she brought her mom a box of chocolates. To Kay's surprise, she noticed there was already a box on the table. When she asked her where they came from, Kay's mom replied, "My boyfriend." It was Kay's wish come true.

Hal treasured Kay's mother. While the caregivers were not thrilled about other romantic encounters between residents, her mother and Hal's love was special and brought a smile to their lips.

Sadly, Hal passed before Kay's mom. One afternoon, shortly after he died, Kay was talking to her mother and noticed that she wasn't looking at her but rather at something else in the room that was not visible to Kay. At this point, Kay's mother was non-verbal, but they could still communicate just fine.

The hospice nurse had told Kay it was common for people in transition to see loved ones, so she asked her if someone was in the room with them. Kay's mom nodded yes with a smile. Kay asked if it was her father, and her mom shook her head no. She then asked if it was someone who made her happy. Kay's mom again nodded yes. Finally, she asked, "Is it Hal?" Her mom's face lit up, and she vigorously nodded YES!

Kay's mother passed away shortly after that visit from her love, Hal, three months after his death.

Robin: Little Messages from Dad

My friend Robin's father Joel was 87, and in poor health, yet no matter what happened to him, he always had a positive attitude. He died during the Covid pandemic in 2020, and Robin told me what kept her going was receiving little messages from the spirit world that keep them connected.

For example, one night, Robin found herself missing her father terribly. Although she seldom watched television, this particular night she decided to turn it on. One of Joel and Robin's favorite shows to watch together was *Jeopardy*, and at that exact moment, she heard one of the contestants say, "Be of good cheer." During his last phase, Joel had become wheelchair-bound, and when Robin would visit him at the Motion Picture Home, he would routinely say, "Be of good cheer." She felt he was still right there with her.

James: The Gift of Love & Compassion

Ed, my friend James' father, was a 95-year-old, non-verbal man with impaired vision and hearing. One day, James got a call that Ed had a stroke. He rushed from Los Angeles to Chicago to be by his side. When he arrived, James discovered his dad was now paralyzed, except for a repetitive arm movement on his left side. Ed's arm would bend at the elbow, his hand would move down to his side, and then back up to his shoulder, neck, and chin. This uncontrollable pattern would repeat several times a minute.

Despite the involuntary movement, doctors told James his father was no longer responsive. However, when James sat with Ed, he saw that even though his father was lying there silently with his eyes closed, he was still processing information and communicating with him.

Like other father-son relationships, many things were unspoken between them, especially when it came to feelings and emotional experiences. James had suffered from depression in his teens and had lied to his father, fearing a tough-love response, like a stern, uncompassionate drill sergeant. James later learned that his father had suffered similar feelings growing up, but he had never admitted his secret to James.

In those final days, as James sat there with Ed, his thoughts and honest feelings about their journey together flowed freely. He wanted to make amends for not telling his father the truth about his depression. Once he admitted his secret and apologized, Ed miraculously opened his eyes, and James felt his father's complete love and compassion. It was a long-awaited moment of forgiveness and completion between a father and son — a shared emotional relatedness.

James also told his father about each of his close friends, how much he loved them, and what a wonderful life he had. He was sitting beside Ed, gently connecting with him by resting his hand on his chest.

As James continued to share other intimate details about his feelings, his father's body language shifted, and the repetitive arm movement stopped. It was the first time his arm had been still since James arrived. Suddenly, Ed reached for James' hands and slid them both over his heart, where they remained in stillness for several minutes. Again, Ed opened his eyes in acknowledgment. James said he felt his father's gesture was like a big, loving hug, and at that moment, all of the resentments of the past dissolved. (The memories may remain but were no longer resentments.)

Even though I was on the West Coast, I had been receiving subtle messages from Ed periodically while James was there sitting bedside. But the strongest transmission came when James described this experience. I could feel Ed's love and presence in the room with me.

As we spoke, I was looking at a beautiful poster hanging on my wall of a mandala created by a group of monks. I purchased two copies of the print when I attended an event where they prepared a traditional meal for myself and some friends on sacred land overlooking the California coast. The poster had been securely hanging on my wall for many years with no incident. However, as James relayed his touching intimate story of connection, the poster fell off the wall and landed with the printed side facing upward. The inscription read: "The Art of Love and Compassion."

At first, I missed the significance of the message and rehung the poster. But each time I spoke to James, it fell off the wall again. Once I realized it was a message from Ed to James, I told him about it.

After Ed's passing, the picture fell off the wall one more time. A few days later, I came across the extra print of the poster and heard Ed ask, "Would you please give this to my son in appreciation for our time together?"

I obliged Ed and gave it to James for Christmas. My print has remained secure on the wall ever since.

Walter: A Guardian Angel Grandma

Walter takes the train to work, where he has a high-pressure job as a doctor at a hospital. One Monday, when he got on the train during the Covid pandemic, only one empty seat was left. After he sat down, he was surprised to find that sitting across from him was the nurse who had cared for his grandmother during her transition — someone he hadn't seen since she passed away.

The nurse shared how much he had loved working for Walter's grandmother and showed him photos he had taken of her that were still on his phone. Walter said it was such a wonderful conversation and how much he loved seeing those pictures! As he was getting off the train, he realized that it was exactly one year to the day that his grandmother had died.

Walter had been struggling with the demands of his job since the pandemic began and was having trouble sleeping. He had broken down several times that week at work before testing positive for the coronavirus on Thursday. Walter was immediately sent home to quarantine for two weeks.

Later that day, he got a phone call from his boss, who said that if his numbers were down over the weekend, he would no longer be considered contagious and should return to work on Monday. Walter was furious at the thought that the hospital was being so reckless with both his health and the welfare of others and wasn't sure what to do about it.

Minutes later, one of his ex-colleagues who worked at a different local hospital called to let him know that a position had just opened up and expressed that it was a low-stress, wonderful place to work. His friend invited him to apply when he was out of quarantine.

As Walter shared this story with me, he said that after meeting the nurse on the train, he felt sure that his grandmother was letting him know that she was beautifully watching over him by opening new doors for him to bring balance and happiness back into his life.

Tiffany: A Little Humor

My daughter and I met Tiffany when she was 14 at a ranch where I used to keep my horse. We had always known Tiffany as an upbeat, happy teen with a wonderful sense of humor. She loved playing tricks on everyone at the ranch, especially her father. What we didn't know was that Tiffany had frequent migraines, but her doctors felt they were fairly normal for her age. Then one day, Tiffany suddenly died from a brain aneurysm.

Tiffany's family was Buddhist, and her funeral was held at a beautiful temple downtown. The ceremony was unlike anything I had experienced; it was very formal, and the speakers were eloquent. Hundreds of people were in attendance, and Tiffany's family had arranged for a police escort to lead the caravan of cars from the temple, across several freeways, to a cemetery in the San Fernando Valley, about forty minutes away.

As we patiently waited for the motorcade to begin, Danielle and I discussed how devastating her loss was for so many, yet we felt that Tiffany wouldn't have wanted us all to be so sad. Shortly after our conversation, we both noticed some commotion around the front of the caravan line. The hearse carrying Tiffany's body had a dead battery, and the funeral company had sent another hearse to give it a jump start.

Finally, they got it started, and everyone in the procession shifted their vehicles back into gear. But seconds later, the hearse sputtered and turned off again. My daughter and I giggled at the thought that Tiffany was playing one of her jokes to lighten the mood. We weren't the only ones finding humor in the situation — everyone else was also laughing in their cars.

Next, the funeral company transferred her body from the dead hearse to the one they'd used to jumpstart it. To our amusement, that one wouldn't start either. Eventually, they brought in a third hearse, and it fired right up. My daughter and I both agreed that Tiffany was enjoying the spectacle and quite amused.

When the spirits come ringing …

A friend recently sent me a link to a TikTok clip of Nurse Penny (@nurse_penny), a hospice nurse who answers questions for people related to death through her experiences. I loved this story and wanted to share it with you.

Nurse Penny was working the night shift at a care center where they kept the doors locked at night. The nurses carried pagers that would ring when someone buzzed the doorbell. One night, the bell rang when Nurse Penny was on shift, and when she went to the front door, no one was there. She told one of the other nurses what happened, who laughed and said, "Ah, that happens all the time; it's just the spirits coming to get the patients." Sure enough, moments later, one of our patients died.

BABA
A GRANDMOTHER'S CONFUSED SOUL

Vignette Ten

♥

This story is a little different from the rest — sometimes the very human "spirit" of desire can prolong a person's transition by confusing their soul, especially when they are elderly. "Baba," the grandmother of my client Natalie, was one of those people. I had been holistically caring for her since she was in her early nineties.

Natalie invited me to Baba's bedside when she was in transition, to help assess her. When I arrived, Baba was extremely uncomfortable, very restless, and by all appearances already deeply integrating with the other side. It was evident that her 101-year-old body was well past its expiration date.

Natalie explained that her family was in denial about the reality of the situation and wasn't yet willing to discuss hospice care. I felt this conflict between the family members was confusing her grandmother and she didn't understand it was time to let go.

About an hour into our visit, Baba's 80+-year-old doctor arrived. He was seductively charming and came in with enormous energy — like a rooster in a hen house. This charismatic doctor leaned in to give Baba a big kiss and announced, "You look beautiful today, my dear." As frail and pale as she was, she blushed like a teenager. He told her that she'd be up and about in no time.

At that moment, I realized there was much more happening than just the family dynamics keeping her alive. I could see that her doctor wasn't there to support her transition, but instead was trying to prolong Baba's life — despite the reality of her age and physical condition. These were a lot of conflicting messages for a dying elderly woman to process.

Unfortunately, it took another month and a lot of actions on the family's part after finally coming to terms with the reality before Baba finally was able to let go and rest peacefully. One night she simply waited until everyone went home to take her last breath — alone.

RIC & KAREN
A HOLLYWOOD ENDING

Vignette Eleven

Ric's story of completion was something out of a Hollywood movie — a "message from beyond" with a twist. This first-of-a-kind (for me) experience gave me a whole different understanding of the depth of a soul's abilities.

Karen and I met in the early '80s when she and I worked for Norman Lear at his corporate offices in Century City. She was only there for a short period of time before moving to the studio. Ten years later I was reintroduced to Karen at a friend's party. She became a client and, over time, a friend.

A few years into our friendship, I received an invitation from Karen's father, Ric, to a milestone birthday party he was hosting for her. I hadn't yet met him, but I had heard stories about him over the years. Ric was an actor and sounded like a real character.

Everyone was already seated when I arrived at the restaurant, and the only empty chair was next to Ric. He was a large, handsome Italian man wearing an expensive sports coat with slacks and comfortable walking shoes. I could tell immediately by the climate at the table that it would be an interesting evening. Ric and I hit it off right away, swapping stories about ridiculous escapades within the entertainment industry, and the night proved to be quite enjoyable.

212

Ric had a lot of health issues and physical limitations and needed full-time care to help with his daily routines. Over time, as his body continued to deteriorate, he relied on his daughter's help with his fan-based business and in maintaining his affairs. Karen knew that I had taken care of my folks in their last chapter, so she would periodically call upon me for guidance in navigating her challenges with her father.

Eventually, Ric's kidneys and liver started failing, and Karen moved him to a local hospital. She asked if I would come to the hospital and give her my opinion about the situation, and I agreed. When I arrived, Ric was happy to see me and clearly remembered our conversation at Karen's birthday party. His overall health was hard to read because he was still fully awake, expressing his wishes coherently. I suggested Karen wait and see what happens over the next few days.

The doctors' and nurses' jobs are to heal and keep their patients alive, so they wanted to perform additional tests while continuing their routine dialysis treatment. Ric agreed, and Karen's job was to simply be there and support his decisions.

About a week later, the rest of his organs had begun to shut down, and Karen again asked if I could stop by to assess his status. When I arrived this time, Ric was resting with his eyes closed. I brought my boyfriend, Dave, along with me, and he sat next to Karen at one end of the room. I took a seat at the foot of Ric's bed. I connected to his energy as Karen and Dave spoke quietly to each other.

Suddenly Ric opened his eyes, looked into mine, and said, "Rosie's here, and she says hello." My stepmother's nickname was Rosie, so I immediately knew he had already moved into a different phase of his process. I told him she was a great person to help him integrate, and he said, "I know," before drifting back off.

I continued to visit daily, having similar intimate energetic moments with Ric. Eventually, the doctors told Karen it was time to make arrangements to move him into hospice. The thought of finding the right place to move her father was so overwhelming to her that I suggested she go home, get some rest, meditate, and see what guidance the universe might offer her.

The following morning, Karen called and excitedly told me she had thought of the perfect place to move him — the Motion Picture Home in Woodland Hills. It was a brilliant idea, and after 24 hours of calls and pleading with management (and a little universal support), a room opened up for Ric. It was the miracle that they both needed.

Karen scheduled the transport for that afternoon and arranged for us to be there to greet him. As they rolled Ric down the hallway, he gave us a big smile, grabbed our hands, and repeatedly thanked us. He was so happy and felt so comforted in being welcomed into this final perfect resting place.

I knew then it would just be a matter of hours, or maybe a day before Ric would pass. They put him in a bright private room with a sliding door that looked out onto a lovely patio area with a table and chairs. Once Ric settled in, I sat with Karen and another friend on the patio, where the two of them told wonderful stories about her dad's entertaining life while he peacefully slept. It was a great honoring of his spirit and accomplishments, and we left the door open so he could hear us.

When I walked in to say goodbye, Ric briefly opened his eyes and thanked me again for my help. As I left, I knew it would be the last time I'd see him. My heart was so full of joy because he was so happy. I leaned in and whispered, "It's time to let go." Ric replied, "I know. Thank you."

The following morning, I got a call from Karen, and she was crying. When she arrived at the home, two different nurses told her that Ric's wife had visited earlier that morning. They had each commented on the woman's unique beauty. Karen was somewhat baffled since Ric had been single for over twenty years, and his ex-wife (her mother) lived in another state. When she asked the nurses to describe the woman, they both said she was beautiful and wore a long white dress. Interestingly, they were describing Ric's mother, who had passed decades ago.

This was the first time I had heard of two different people corroborating an inter-dimensional sighting of the same spirit walking the halls at different moments — a spirit friend, family member, or a stranger from the other side coming to greet and support their journey home across that threshold.

When Karen went in to join her father, he told her that his mother was there and it was time for him to go. He held his hands out and called to his Italian mother — "A ma, a ma." A few minutes later, a light appeared in the room as Ric took his last breath.

It was an expressive, welcoming transition after a long, at times turbulent, father-daughter relationship. Thankfully, they could share that special moment between them as he crossed over — both with affectionate hearts.

CHAPTER 11

FRIENDS' STORIES:
BEING OF SERVICE TO LOVED ONES

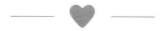

"Even when I think I have nothing to offer someone or find myself in a situation where I feel my hands are empty, I can still give people the most precious thing: my time and undivided attention."
~ James Pluta

The following stories were written by three of my friends — Aimee, James, and Mimi — who were willing to share their personal experiences supporting their loved ones in their last phase. I chose these stories because I thought they were interesting examples of how being of service can look, about becoming our best self, processing fear, forgiving oneself, and completing.

Aimee: *God's Forgiveness*

I am my father's daughter. My dad passed away years ago, and I still think of him daily. He taught me, among many other things, wilderness survival skills. He was prepared for anything. We would set out on a hike in the morning on a gorgeous summer day, and he'd pack a rain slicker, Duct-tape, tissues, Band-Aids, a fresh pair of socks, Moleskin for blisters, a wool hat, and a Ziploc bag, just in case. He made us do the same.

We thought he was crazy, but, sure enough, it paid off. Once my family was caught in a downpour and then, hours later, a hailstorm. From then on, my siblings and I were always grateful to have all of the necessary survival things for our comfort in our backpacks.

My dad never had, nor gave us, the fancy expensive gear. Simple was good enough for him. Less was more. And today, when I look at the big purse I carry around (like a suitcase), people ask me, "What could possibly be in there?"

I always laugh and think of my dad smiling down on me ... because, in a pinch, those people are equally as glad that I have all the essentials for emergencies.

I live in Los Angeles with my husband and two kids. Dad lived in Alabama with my stepmother, Denise, who lovingly cared for him until the end. I loved my father and traveled cross-country often while he was healthy and active. I was equally involved during his 12-year dance with illness, supporting him in everything from making lifestyle changes to seeing doctors, healers, and physical therapists. We would go as a family to visit him, and I would go alone, often thinking it would be my last trip, but he just kept holding on.

At first, Denise and I had our differences about his caregiving, which always bothered my father. However, at some point, she said, "I don't know, we're just going to have to learn to come together and trust each other."

Truthfully, I didn't always trust her, but I trusted God. And over time, I softened my behavior and began to find that trust. Ultimately, I was really grateful we were a team, and she was always there for him (and me).

Denise and I often wondered why letting go was so hard for him. After much reflection and many conversations with him, we concluded that it was most likely about something that had happened when he was in the service (Marines).

Dad told Denise he wasn't sure if God could forgive him for what he had done. As a devout Christian and a very spiritual man, he feared he wouldn't go to heaven. Thankfully, Denise and their minister were able to help him process these feelings with deep conversations and prayer, as they walked him through his "dark night of the soul."

I believe that in my father's final days, he knew God forgave him because once he could trust that he was going to heaven, he began to relax and find a sense of inner peace. Shortly after that, he stopped eating, and his body began to shut down.

Around that time, our church was going on a retreat in the mountains, and I really wanted to go with my husband and kids. It had been such a stressful time for all of us, and we needed some bonding time. I was conflicted about whether to go see my father and help Denise or take this time with my spiritual group and immediate California family.

Denise assured me that she had everything under control, and my dad encouraged me to go and get the rest I needed. I was in agony over the decision but eventually decided to go on the retreat. We spoke on the phone before the trip, and I had also written letters of gratitude to him and Denise and mailed both of them before leaving.

The Retreat & The Universe's Support

As fate would have it, the retreat took place in the mountains where there was virtually no cell service. However, I still found comfort in sleeping with my cell phone by my bed in case, by some miracle, it would work if there were any changes in his condition over the weekend.

Late Friday night, while dozing off, I thought I heard my phone buzz … could it be? Yes, it was Denise reporting that Dad was extremely restless and said he was ready to go. I was shocked that she had gotten through.

Then on Saturday night, she called again to let me know that his body was officially shutting down. Again, the call came through in an area that supposedly had no cell service. I was so grateful … I suggested she have her nurse friend come over to sit with them that night.

Denise agreed and also called their minister and several other friends to come and support the process. They all graciously accepted and surrounded them both in their love.

On Sunday morning, as I was preparing to lead a final faith circle activity, the phone rang through one more time. "Your father has just taken his final breath," Denise said softly.

I felt such a sense of relief … Yes, it was a great loss, yet I had already done so much of my grieving leading up to this moment that I truly felt at peace.

I hung up the phone and walked into the main building, where my friends and faith community awaited me. All of the people in the room were from our church of 20 years, a place where my husband and I were married and had baptized our children and so much more. This was my safe community.

The words flowed out of me: "I just received some news… my father passed away." There was a deep and embracing sigh from the group as they all gathered around me, bathing me in the essence of their divine love with one of the biggest connected hugs I have ever received. I cried and allowed myself to be held. I was exactly where I needed to be at that moment in the open and loving arms of my friends. I later found out that at the same time, Denise was surrounded by her group of friends and family, embraced in her own circle of support. We were both in our perfect space in time.

Later that day, my family and I drove down the mountain, and I knew deep in my heart that everything was okay. Denise and I had shepherded Daddy to the other side in an amazing way. We had done it together. My father never got the letter I wrote him in his physical life, but I am certain that it was delivered to him in that other realm. Denise received hers with the deepest gratitude.

There is no perfect way to do life, and there is no perfect way to do death. Dad took it slowly and methodically, just like he took every aspect of his life. God was with us every step of the way in walking him home. I talk to Denise weekly, and we constantly email, text, and write. She is one of my closest friends today. And my dad is smiling down at us. He will always be with me in my heart. Always.

James: *Meeting My Best Self*

Ken was my best friend of seventeen years and my sponsor in Alcoholics Anonymous (AA). He was a kind, humble, and generous man who taught me so much about communication, friendships, life, and how to fully trust another human being. Ken was always there when I needed him giving me his full attention and listening with deep respect. He was a living example of who I wanted to be and became one of the most significant people in my life.

One day Ken asked if we could meet for lunch. When we met, I knew something was wrong from the palpable sense of trepidation in his voice. "My doctor has found a tumor on one of my kidneys."

My initial response was one of deflecting reality. While the news shook me, I knew I would have to hold a steadfast position of strength and safety for him. However, as I connected to the truth of his cancer diagnosis, I was also confronted with my deeper fears. I was not ready to lose Ken.

In the following days, I remembered a promise I had made to another friend when someone we knew passed away the year before — always to let those we care about know how we feel about them while they are alive. There were so many people I loved that I had never told before they passed. When they were sick, I never even thought of asking how I could be of service to them.

Ken had given so freely to me; this was my chance to learn how to show up and be there for him. I wanted to give him the best of me, but I didn't yet know that part of myself. I even wondered if I could be that kind of person.

Giving Back & Fulfilling Dreams

Thankfully, Ken's initial bout with cancer was resolved by removing a kidney and chemotherapy treatments. The whole process was pretty straightforward, and his recovery was fairly easy. He really didn't require much more than some emotional support at that time, which I, and many others, gladly provided.

Nonetheless, for that instant, we were all reminded of how short life is and how we never know when our time will be up. I also realized how important it is to live fully in every moment, being present, happy, and enjoying life, especially when new opportunities arise.

Since Ken was a true workingman, he had lived a fairly predictable life, rarely traveling for pleasure or seeing much of the world. As a producer of concert documentaries, I, on the other hand, had the opportunity to travel extensively, capturing iconic popular musical history, something most people have only dreamt about, including Ken.

A year after Ken's reported clean bill of health, I took on a project in London, filming a concert at the Royal Albert Hall. I would be there for a few weeks prepping for the four-night shoot that would have fifteen cameras simultaneously videotaping throughout. All of the tapes would then need to be hand-carried back to Los Angeles to meet our release deadline.

I spontaneously asked Ken if he wanted to work for me and take an all-expense-paid trip to London. With a mixture of fear of the unknown and the excitement of riding a bike for the first time without the training wheels, he said yes. A month later, we were in London.

It was an unforgettable trip for both of us and despite my work schedule, we were able to spend quality time with each other. Ken was so happy and grateful, and my heart was filled with joy to have been able to give him this opportunity.

Cancer — Round Two

New cancer cells began metastasizing to different areas in his body the following year. I watched as the doctors played Whack-a-Mole chasing it around with different treatments. I knew this time his longevity was now in jeopardy, and I could no longer deflect or dance around this reality — and neither could he.

A core group of Ken's friends and I made his care our priority and set up a daily rotation of duties between us. He could no longer work and eventually moved in with his daughter, who looked in on him between her classes and job. We took turns taking him grocery shopping, to AA meetings, and transporting him to his medical appointments. Ken tried both traditional and experimental treatments over the next couple of years, but the cancer was relentless. As a community, we emotionally and physically supported him throughout.

During one of Ken's appointments, when we were waiting for the doctor, both of us noticed the headline on one of the magazines that read, "The End is Near." Moments later, the doctor came in and confirmed that Ken had six months at most left to live — a prognosis that shook us both.

Ken decided that six months of life shared with friends and family without the drugs was far more meaningful to him than extra time with painful treatment. Our support team for him grew between his battles, wins, and setbacks over the next six months.

Sunday Pizza Parties

When Ken moved into his last phase, I wanted to do something special to uplift everyone's spirits, and our Sunday afternoon pizza parties were born. Growing up in the Chicago suburbs, I often bragged about how we had the best pizza in the world. That's when I began ordering pizzas from my favorite Chicago restaurant, which arrived frozen on Sunday mornings in time to cook up for our afternoon parties. Everyone loved the pizza and looked forward to our gatherings, especially Ken. There was so much love around him.

In his last few weeks, two things happened. First, on one of my visits, Ken called me into his room and asked that I close the door behind me. The time had come that he would need 24-hour care, and his family couldn't afford it. They were talking about moving him to a hospice facility. Ken was upset and crystal clear that whatever time he had left was about his quality of life and comfort. He expressed how happy he was living with his daughter and he wasn't emotionally ready to deal with a change. He loved looking out the window and watching the sunset against the Santa Monica mountains with the famous Hollywood sign. Ken asked if I could help ensure his last wish of staying there.

At that moment, I knew that even if I had to fund the situation myself, I would make it happen for this incredible man who had given so much of himself to me (and so many others.) Fortunately, after speaking with a few of the other men, we were able to 'pass the hat' and share the expense of his overnight nurse care.

Second, on another night, when I arrived, he was sitting in his room alone, very focused and doing an interesting movement with his hands. When I asked what he was doing, he said, "I'm sewing." When he was done with his mending, he handed it to me and asked that I put his project in a safe place for him to continue work on later. I obliged him and showed him where I was putting his imaginary work.

A few minutes later, he looked out the window and began talking to what he referred to as the "Knuckleheads," a nickname he jokingly called his sponsees in AA. He imagined them on his patio, peering in his window from outside in the dark. When he finished conversing with them, he appeared to feel relaxed and complete.

I interpreted both actions as if he were mending something, like incomplete relationships, and then saying goodbye to his friends (or perhaps they were friends there to greet him). While I didn't fully understand what was happening, and some might have considered this a hallucination, I felt like I was witnessing something extraordinary.

Ken passed away three weeks after his full-time care began and a few nights after the evening of his completion of tying up loose ends and visiting with his spirit friends in the comfort of his room — a room with a magnificent view.

The Gift(s) of Giving

Ultimately, my experience of being of service and showing up for Ken brought with it many invaluable unexpected gifts. It taught me about what really matters in life: simplicity. Even when I think I have nothing to offer someone or find myself in a situation where I feel my hands are empty, I can still give people the most precious thing: my time and undivided attention.

My experience with Ken opened my heart and showed me that I could give of myself without question through acts of kindness and experience a sense of wholeness and completeness in my relationship with someone while they are still here. I met that best part of myself, and I was able to experience unconditional love.

Mimi: *Saint Anthony's Prayer*

My father was seventy years old when he was diagnosed with prostate cancer. His doctor recommended radiation, but my father balked and asked how long he might live if he didn't do it. The doctor told him eight years, give or take. My father replied, "Then I don't need radiation because I will die anyway when I am seventy-eight, just like my stepfather!" Fortunately, his particular cancer was slow-moving, and my father was able to carry on with his life.

My biological grandfather died in his early thirties when my dad was only seven. Daddy didn't have much information about his father's death, just that he went to work one day and never came home. I believe that sudden loss was when my dad developed his love for Saint Anthony, my Italian grandmother's favorite saint.

Saint Anthony's prayer was said to give hope — a promise of finding lost things. This saint is usually depicted holding the Christ child in his arms, and I think my father yearned to find his father and be held like that. His connection with Saint Anthony and the prayer was so strong that he typed it out on onion skin paper and insisted that we learn and recite it every Tuesday as well. I always kept it folded in my wallet for safekeeping and easy access.

God's Plan - A Quick Exit

Then one morning, I received a call from my father's sister telling me my father had had a mini-stroke. She asked him if he wanted us to come, and he said, "No. I don't want them to see me like this." I spoke to him and said, "Don't be ridiculous," and promptly booked a flight to the East Coast.

When I arrived, I was directed to a wing of the hospital that my dad had helped raise money to build. His name was on a plaque hanging on the wall. It was a good thing I'd moved quickly to get there because he had already experienced another more massive stroke and could no longer speak or move his body.

My sister also flew in, and we sat bedside with him on opposite sides, holding his hands. He started exhaling powerfully, and I told my sister I thought he was trying to express something. She replied, "Stop reading into it, Mimi. Those are just involuntary muscle reflexes." I remained unconvinced.

Whatever was happening, he was extremely uncomfortable. The doctors began to think he might be having a secondary issue, a stomach infection known to be painful, and they wanted to take some X-rays. My sister agreed, but my gut reaction was not to move him, especially if he was dying.

Unfortunately, I was outnumbered. As the assistants transferred my dad to a gurney, he groaned in greater protest, and I felt then that he was trying to speak with his breath. These were NOT involuntary exhalations but attempts to communicate.

We were all standing in the hall, and I tried to orient him to what was happening by reminding him what day of the week it was and the time. I explained that we were there waiting for his turn to have some tests run. I tried to comfort him by smoothing his hair back from his forehead and reassuring him of how much I loved him. My sister leaned in and said, "Daddy, I love you too."

Dad turned his head towards her and exhaled a really long, deep breath. I thought, "That's it. He's going to die right now." Just then, I saw a tear in the corner of his eye.

Throughout my father's life, he used to say that when you cry out of the corner of your eye, you know you are happy. My father and sister's relationship had always been complicated. For him to hear her say these words, for her to mean them, and for him to believe her was a special gift.

I believe that tear was a sign of his happiness. I also think that if we hadn't moved him per my sister's insistence, that exchange and pivotal moment of forgiveness between them might have never happened. It was just another example that everything is happening exactly as it should be.

As I witnessed his anxiety and physical discomfort growing, I wondered if my father had forgotten his sense of faith as he prepared to die. Was he lost and afraid of dying, or a man who may have seen his own behaviors as unforgiving and even sinful at times?

In those moments of not knowing, all I could do was tap into my intuition and upbringing, hoping to access some spiritual intervention to help soothe his anxiety. Through my tears, I commanded, "Call Saint Anthony Daddy. You have the right! You said that prayer every Tuesday your entire life. Call Saint Anthony to come to your aid!" There was a notable shift in his energy, and I believe he called upon this prayer and heard a response because he immediately calmed down.

Finding Peace in Those Final Moments

When he returned from the tests, I could see that he was actively dying. A hospice nun followed closely behind him as my dad continued to strongly exhale. It sounded like he was talking to someone. The nun asked me, "Who do you think he's talking to?" To me, it sounded like he was saying, "Mother." The nun agreed.

Once he heard us acknowledge this encounter, he said, "Father." We asked him if he was seeing his father. After confirmation of his facial expression, the word changed again. This time the word was 'Why?' Knowing his history, I thought that perhaps he was asking why his father had left him. Daddy was quiet, as though he was listening to his father's explanation. My father was a lawyer; he always needed to know why. He wanted to know every detail about the cases he worked on.

A moment later, he said, "All right." I wondered if he had been shown some karmic record of "why." Was his father able to show him how karmic justice had been achieved by his leaving early?

My father said, "Okay, okay, okay. That's right." While I'll never know for sure what he was experiencing during that exchange, I found comfort in my imaging thoughts.

Dad finally seemed to be at peace as he moved into some softer, quiet exhalations. A few moments later, there was another sharp inhalation, and I felt my mother's presence. I was sure that she had come to walk him home to Jesus. My mom had a big God thing going on, and the energy in the room felt like they were being reunited. Then after one last huge, significant, glorious intake of air and an expansive, powerful exhale, he was gone.

I sat there, taking in the vastness of that moment and the essence of the energy of the experience. As the passage of my father's spirit still filled the room, I reflected on his worn body. His feet were scarred and blistered, purple and blue — like old people. I thought to myself, *we should go bearing all our scars proudly.* It's not about, "Don't let them see me like this." There is no shame, but rather testimony to, "I've used this body to the best of my ability, and now I leave it behind for you to know I made yours. And life on earth is holy."

CHAPTER 12

BEAUTIFUL ENDINGS & NEW BEGINNINGS

Florrie & Harvey (an imaginary friend)
Walk Barney Home Together

One of the most touching stories my friend Florrie shared with me the afternoon I interviewed her for Chapter 5, "Creating A Death Plan," was about Barney, the five-year-old son of her dear friends, Pat and Sandy. Barney had cancer, and even though Florrie was managing a literary agency at the time, she decided to take a month off to help support the family.

Florrie visited Barney every day, where she would find him resting on the couch, preparing for his transition. One day she decided to get creative and arrived with her arm extended upward as if she were holding hands with a taller imaginary friend. When Barney asked what Florrie was doing, she told him she had brought her friend Harvey to meet him. When Barney said he couldn't see him, she said, "Well, I can see him, and if I can see him, surely you'll be able to see him."

Barney asked, "What does Harvey look like?" Florrie described him as being a kind and loving big brother, something he had always dreamed of, and then exclaimed, "I can tell that he likes you!"

Barney asked what he should do with Harvey. Florrie replied that Harvey wanted to sit beside him. She suggested that he move over a little bit and make room for Harvey. Barney adjusted his body to accommodate his guest, and the three talked throughout the afternoon. When it came time for Florrie to leave, Barney asked if Harvey could stay.

Surprised by his request, she said, "Sure. You bet. I'll pick him up tomorrow, okay?"

Barney agreed. He was so weak at this point that he could no longer play games with his friends, so at that moment, an imaginary friend was the perfect gift and the best medicine ever.

The following morning, Florrie learned that Barney had been transferred to the hospital, so she quickly headed over to see him. When she walked into his room, she was surprised by what she saw; Barney had positioned himself on one half of the bed to share his space with Harvey, his new special friend. She felt a warming sense of love from this incredibly touching picture. Harvey remained by Barney's side until the day he died. Harvey was the one who walked Barney home.

Florrie had instinctively facilitated this beautiful friendship between the physical and dimensional realms of the two worlds. As she shared this story with me, she told me it was one of the proudest moments and acts of her life.

As I mentioned earlier, Florrie passed away in August 2023. What is so beautiful about this story is that today Florrie and Barney are together again at Westwood Village Memorial Park.

At Florrie's celebration of life, her niece read this story. When she finished, one of the guests, a man named Judson, asked to speak. He started by saying that, like many others, Florrie had adopted him as one of her spiritual kids and how much that relationship meant to him. He then became emotional and, to everyone's surprise, told us that had Barney lived, he would have been his older brother.

Judson had never heard that story about Barney or knew what Florrie had done for his brother and their family. His parents never talked about Barney, and Judson was so grateful to have heard this story about the brother he never met and what that experience had meant to Florrie. It was a beautiful gift for him and all of us.

Feeling Complete & Divine Timing — Sparky

Charles M. Schultz (aka "Sparky"), who brought us Charlie Brown, Snoopy, and the whole Peanuts gang, had written a letter of gratitude to his fans announcing his retirement. This farewell message was to appear in his final comic strip in the Sunday paper on February 13, 2000. Sparky died in his sleep on February 12, 2000 — the night before. This is a beautiful example of someone feeling and being complete.

A Love Story Until the End — Leonard & Marianne

Leonard Cohen was a Canadian singer, songwriter, poet, and novelist ("Hallelujah" is his most famous song). His one true love was a Norwegian woman named Marianne Ihlen. She was his creative muse and inspiration for several of his songs, including

"Bird on the Wire," and "So Long, Marianne." She also appeared on the back cover of Cohen's second album, *Songs from a Room*.

Despite their love for one another, their eight-year romantic relationship ended in 1978. The two of them stayed in touch through letters and, towards the end, emails, always speaking fondly of one another and their love when asked by others.

After Cohen's passing, the final email communication between Ihlen and Cohen was released to the public. As I reflected on them, I felt in my heart that their love and relationship had come full circle in this beautiful story of completion, and I wanted to share it with you.

In the summer of 2016, Cohen received an email from Ihlen's close friend Jan Christian Mollestad, letting him know that Ihlen had been hospitalized with leukemia and was in her final days.

Within hours Cohen wrote back to Mollestad, asking him to tell Ihlen that he would be just a little behind her, close enough to take her hand. He empathized with both of their physical conditions and said that his "eviction notice" would also arrive any day. He acknowledged their love and wished her a safe journey — telling Mollestad to let her know that he would see her down the road shortly.

Two days later, Cohen received an email from Norway letting him know that Ihlen had left this life in her sleep, surrounded by her friends. Thankfully, Ihlen received Cohen's response while she could still talk and laugh in full consciousness. When Mollestad read Cohen's words about him being close enough to take her hand, she lifted her arm as if to reach for his.

In her last moments, Mollestad held her hand and hummed "Bird on the Wire" as she took her last shallow breaths. He later wrote to Cohen:

"And when we left the room after her soul had flown out of the window for new adventures, we kissed her head and whispered your everlasting words. So long, Marianne."

I believe that Cohen's final words to Ihlen were what she was waiting for to feel complete. Leonard Cohen passed away three and a half months later, and I imagine that Marianne was waiting with an extended hand to usher her friend home.

You can view their letters online or learn more about their interesting love story in the beautiful documentary — *Marianne & Leonard: Words of Love.*

♥

A Big, Glorious Sigh — Father Gregory Boyle

In 2018, I witnessed a wonderful conversation between Father Gregory Boyle, founder of *Homeboy Industries* (a gang-intervention, rehabilitation, and re-entry program), and Buddhist teacher, and author, Pema Chödrön at UCLA's Royce Hall in California. Their intimate conversation covered a variety of different aspects of kindness and mindfulness, including around the subject of dying. This is one of the sweet stories Father Greg told about his experience of being with his mother in her final weeks:

"Not long ago, I buried my 89-year-old mother. She was sharp as a tack until the very end. And even though she watched so much MSNBC that she was becoming Rachel Maddow, she wasn't a lick afraid of dying. She would say things like, 'I can't wait to go home.'

She was exuberant and excited about it, 'I've just never done this before.'

In fact, in the days before she died, she would be asleep and suddenly wake up and see me sitting there and say, 'Oh, for crying out loud, I'm still here.' She would be pissed off that she hadn't died yet.

In the last week, when she was in and out of consciousness and would wake up, she'd always lock on to one of us kids (there were eight of us), and with breathless delight, would say, 'You're here.' In the end, it was just the two of us, and she let out this big glorious sigh like she was skydiving. It was wonderful!"

And New Beginnings ...

A Love Story of Two Widowed Geese

A goose named Blossom and her partner Bud lived at the Riverside Cemetery in Iowa. When Bud died, the General Manager noticed how lonely and sad Blossom was, so he decided to post a personal ad for a new partner for her.

It read, "Lonely, widowed domestic goose — Life partner for companionship and occasional shenanigans. Blossom is youthful, adventurous, and lively." To everyone's surprise, Randy and Deb Hoyt, who were also dealing with a lonely widowed goose named Frankie, responded.

A blind date was arranged for Valentine's Day, and Blossom welcomed Frankie with open wings. A match possibly orchestrated from heaven? They live at the Riverside Cemetery, where they are inseparable and enjoy afternoon dips in the lake.

In the end, all any of us really need is LOVE.

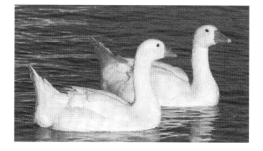

ACKNOWLEDGMENTS

My heart is filled with an abundance of love and gratitude for all those who have contributed to bringing this book to actualization — it takes a village. Every person I have met on this journey has contributed in some way and taught me new lessons. Writing the book was a beautiful vessel that allowed the experiences that lived within me to flow through me onto these pages.

One of the things I am most grateful for is the ability to sit and listen and connect with my intuition with an open heart. In doing so, I was able to hear my friends and family's spirits, who willingly assisted me from the other side in bringing their stories to life. Whoever I was writing about would inevitably pop into my consciousness and become my co-author, keeping me entertained by lending their love, humor, and gratitude. When I would forget specific details, they would enthusiastically remind me what needed to be included — producing spontaneous outbursts of laughter and tears of joy. To those amazing souls and spirits, I say thank you!

I would also like to acknowledge and thank all of the people who so generously opened their hearts and shared their intimately personal stories (you know who you are), as well as the families who gave their blessings for me to share my experience supporting their loved ones as they crossed over — there are no words to convey my deep gratitude!

Thank you to the following inspirational people and organizations for permitting me to use their related insightful personal quotes, excerpts, and stories: Frank Ostaseski, Jan Christian Mollestad, Father Gregory Boyle, Brené Brown, Jeff Kober, Parallax Press for Thich Nhat Hanh, The Fred Rogers Foundation, the Bauerschmidt family, Hospice Nurse Penny (Hawkins Smith), and OSHO International.

I am also grateful to and for …

Alexandra Thompson, "Lexy," my first friend on this earthly plain. Thank you for your lifelong friendship, unconditional love, belief in me, encouragement, inspiration for reading, emotional and outstanding editing support, especially during COVID-19, and endless consulting sessions, which helped nurse me and the book along. I truly could not have done it without you!

Jeff Kober, for generously sharing your wisdom, knowledge, and humor through your weekly gatherings, which help bring this human experience into perspective in such a relatable way. Your invaluable gift of teaching me how to sit with myself and meditate and how to follow that tug of charm has forever enhanced and changed my life. Thank you!

Trudi Roth, for your insightful editing skills, brilliant organizational creativity, and how divinely the universe brought us together to walk this book home together. You have been a wonderful literary midwife. Witnessing your opening to the other realm and the ensuing miracles have filled my heart with joy! Thank you for your enthusiasm and affirmation and for reminding me that this isn't simply a book about consciously living and dying but also about a movement in life.

Last but certainly not least, my daughter, Danielle, for your continued support in all I do and for unconditionally loving and honoring my uniqueness.

Thank you all — I am forever grateful!

RESOURCES

Chapter 2: Meditation: *Finding Stillness in Life to Prepare for Death*

Resources to learn more about meditation (These are just a few to get you started):

- HeartMath (Heart Brain Communication) – HeartMath.org

Books for Adults:

- *You Are Here: Discovering the Magic of the Present Moment* by Thich Nhat Hanh
- *Total Meditation: Practices in Living the Awakened Life* by Deepak Chopra
- *Wherever You Go, There You Are: Mindfulness meditation in Everyday Life* by Jon Kabat-Zinn
- *How to Meditate: A Practical Guide to Making Friends with Your Mind* by Pema Chödrön
- *Mindfulness in Plain English* by Bhante Gunaratana
- *Journey of Awakening: A Meditator's Guidebook* by Ram Dass
- *The Untethered Soul: The Journey Beyond Yourself* by Michael A. Singer
- *The Power of Now: A Guide to Spiritual Enlightenment* by Eckhart Tolle
- *Embracing Bliss: 108 Daily Meditations by* Jeff Kober
- *Practical Meditation for Beginners: 10 Days to a Happier, Calmer You* by Benjamin W. Decker

Books for Children:

- *Just Breathe: Meditation, Mindfulness, Movement, and More* by Mallika Chopra
- *Sensational Meditation for Children: Child-Friendly Meditation Techniques Based on the Five Senses* by Sarah Wood Vallely
- *Healing Breath: A Guided Meditation Through Nature for Kids* by William Meyer

Online and in-person resources and events:

- Jeff Kober Meditation (Jeff-Kober.com): Jeff Kober hosts free intro talks and weekly online group meditations and knowledge meetings in the Vedic tradition.
- Deepak Chopra (Deepakchopra.com): Learn more about Deepak Chopra through a wide variety of offerings at the intersection of spirituality and science (podcasts, courses, books).
- Tara Brach (Tarabrach.com): Explore teacher Tara Brach's contributions to Western Buddhism, including groups, courses, meditations, and talks.
- The Neutral Mind Meditation (Theneutralmindonline.com): The Neutral Mind Meditation Center's founder, Jenna Tighe, hosts free weekly online group meditations and rounding sessions (an advanced version of Vedic Meditation).
- The Shakti Sisters (Theshaktisisters.com): The Shakti Sisters, Diana Charkalis and Trudi Roth, host free online intro talks and weekly group meditations in Vedic tradition.
- The Buddhist Centre (Thebuddhistcentre.com): Explore a variety of free resources, including meditations, articles, and talks.

- The Buddhist Society (Thebuddhistsociety.org): Provides a range of classes and courses in the Buddha's teachings, as well as instruction in Buddhist meditation and daily life practice.
- Lion's Roar (Lionsroar.com): An online magazine and media resource dedicated to sharing Buddhist wisdom for our modern times.
- Light Watkins (Lightwatkins.com): Online community, The Happiness Insider; Holds inspirational challenges and conducts meditation retreats.
- Colors in Motion (Colorsinmotion.com): Relaxing and calming video content for meditative experiences.

Meditation Apps: A variety of free and paid options in each app; available in the App Store and on Google Play

- Headspace (Headspace.com)
- Calm (Calm.com)
- Waking Up (WakingUp.com)
- Insight Timer (Insighttimer.com)
- Healthy Minds Innovations (hmInnovations.org)
- Mindfulness (Mindfulness.com)

Chapter 3: Making Friends with Death

Emotional Freedom Technique – EFT

The following three resources offer free educational tools, apps, and videos to explore.

- Thetappingsolution.com
- Thetappingsolutionfoundation.org
- EFTuniverse.com

Bach Flower Essence Remedies

The following books are good resources for understanding the benefits of flower essences, how to use them, and which ones might be best for your specific emotional imbalance.

- *Bach Flowers For Children – Raising Emotionally Healthy Children Without Drugs* by Kathy Arnos (available at kathyarnos.com)
  This is a great book for beginners, and it's a relatively quick read (45 pages). It teaches the reader about the 38 different remedies and how to use them. While it's a helpful handbook for parents, the information is applicable to people of all ages. (Animals, too!)
- *Bach Flower Therapy – The Complete Approach* by Mechthild Scheffer
  This book is a more comprehensive version of the previous book, *Bach Flowers For Children*.
- *Flower Essence Repertory: A Comprehensive Guide to the Flower Essences –Researched by Dr. Edward Bach and the Flower Essence Society* by Patricia Kaminski and Richard Katz
- A book for serious students, *Flower Essence Repertory* includes the Bach flowers, known as the English flowers, as well as information about the many additional flowers that have been researched and developed over the last 50 years.

For additional information about Bach flowers, visit FesFlowers.com and BachRemedies.com.

Essential Oils and Aromatherapy for Fears
- *The Complete Book of Essential Oils & Aromatherapy* by Valerie Ann Worwood

- *Aromatherapy for the Healthy Child* by Valerie Ann Worwood
- *End-of-Life Care with Essential Oils: Your Guide to Compassionate Care for Loved Ones and Their Caregivers* by Dr. Scott A. Johnson
- *Aromatherapy for Beginners: The Complete Guide to Getting Started with Essential Oils* by Anne Kennedy

Resources for Adults:

The following books offer an introduction to understanding death:

- *On Life after Death* by Elisabeth Kübler-Ross, M.D.
- *Being Mortal: Medicine and What Matters in the End* by Atul Gawande
- *The Five Invitations: Discovering What Death Can Teach Us About Living Fully* by Frank Ostaseski
- *Who Dies? An Investigation of Conscious Living and Conscious Dying* by Stephen Levine and Ondrea Levine
- *The Tibetan Book of Living and Dying* by Sogyal Rinpoche
- *Let's Talk About Death (Over Dinner): An Invitation and Guide to Life's Most Important Conversation* by Michael Hebb
- *Embracing the End of Life: A Journey into Dying & Awakening* by Patt Lind-Kyle, MA
- *The Places That Scare You: A Guide to Fearlessness in Difficult Times* by Pema Chödrön
- *Comfortable with Uncertainty: 108 Teachings on Cultivating Fearlessness and Compassion* by Pema Chödrön
- *Fear: Essential Wisdom for Getting Through the Storm* by Thich Nhat Hanh

- *Letting Go: The Pathway of Surrender* by David R. Hawkins, M.D., Ph.D
- *What If This is Heaven?: How Our Cultural Myths Prevent Us from Experiencing Heaven on Earth* and *Dying To Be Me: My Journey from Cancer, to Near Death, to True Healing* by Anita Moorjani
- *Power vs. Force* by David R. Hawkins, M.D., Ph.D. – Includes Vibrational Frequencies of Emotion, Map of Consciousness Chart

Tools for facing our mortality:

- Alua Arthur, death doula and founder of Going with Grace (Goingwithgrace.com) speaks about fears and death: "I Help People Die for A Living" on the Refinery29 YouTube channel
- Let's talk about death (social groups) —creating social change through live events, and support resources that encourage meaningful conversations, preparation, and connection:
- Death Over Dinner (Deathoverdinner.org) (lifeoverdinner.com) (generationsoverdinner.com)
- Death Cafe (Deathcafe.com)
- End Well (Endwellproject.com)

Resources for Children:

Fortunately, there are many wonderful books and animated films, such as Disney/Pixar's *Soul* and *Coco*, to use as teaching tools to initiate an age-appropriate dialog with children about death. The following books can help teach kids (and adults) about how to identify and process their feelings.

A series of books by Mallika Chopra:

- *Just Be You: Ask Questions, Set Intentions, Be Your Special Self, and More* (Ages: 8-10)
- *Just Feel: How to Be Stronger, Happier, Healthier, and More* (Ages: 8-12)
- *My Body is a Rainbow: The Color of My Feelings* (Ages: 4-8)

Other authors:

- *The Invisible String* by Patrice Karst (Ages: 3-7)
- *What is Death?* By Etan Boritzer (Ages: 6-11)
- *Lifetimes: The Beautiful Way to Explain Death to Children* by Bryan Mellonie and Robert Ingpen (Ages: 3-6)
- *Gorilla Thumps and Bear Hugs: A Tapping Solution Children's Story* by Alex Ortner (Ages: 4-10)
- *What is Given from the Heart* by Patricia C. McKissack (Ages: 4-8)

Chapter 4: Understanding The Cycle of Life: *Birth, Life, Death*

Books/*Organization:

- *How We Live is How We Die* by Pema Chödrön
- *Life's Lessons: Two Experts on Death & Dying Teach Us About the Mysteries of Life & Living by* Elisabeth Kübler-Ross, M.D. and David Kessler
- *The Shift: Taking Your Life from Ambition to Meaning* by Dr. Wayne W. Dyer
- *Journey of the Heart: The Path of Conscious Love* by John Welwood, Ph.D.

- *The Power of Unconditional Love: 21 Guidelines for Beginning, Improving and Changing Your Most Meaningful Relationships* by Ken Keyes, Jr.
- *Anatomy of the Spirit: The Seven Stages of Power and Healing* by Caroline Myss, Ph.D.
- *Dissolving The Ego, Realizing The Self: Contemplations from the Teachings of David R. Hawkins, M.D., Ph.D.*
- *Be Here Now* by Ram Dass
- *Loving What Is: Four questions that can change your life* by Byron Katie
- *A Return to Love: Reflections on the Principles of "A Course in Miracles"* by Marianne Williamson
- *Rising Strong: How the Ability to Reset Transforms the Way We Live, Love, Parent, and Lead* by Brené Brown
- *Waking Up in Winter: In Search of What Really Matters at Midlife* by Cheryl Richardson
- *Wisdom @ Work: The Making of a Modern Elder* and *Learning to Love Midlife: 12 Reasons Why Life Gets Better with Age* by Chip Conley
- *Soul Retrieval: Mending the Fragmented Self* by Sandra Ingerman
- *Journey of Souls: Case Studies of Life Between Lives* by Michael Newton, Ph.D.
- *The Secret Life of the Unborn Child: How You Can Prepare Your Baby for a Happy, Healthy Life* by Thomas Verny, M.D.
- *Communing with the Spirit of Your Unborn Child: A Practical Guide to Intimate Communication with Your Unborn or Infant Child* by Dawson Church
- *Prenatal Psychology 100 Years: A Journey in Decoding How Our Prenatal Experience Shapes Who We Become!* by Olga Gouni, Ludwig Janus, Thomas Verny, M.D., Grigori Brekhman, Jon RG Turner, Troya GN Turner, Dejan

Rakovic, Arthur Janov (Author), Michel Odent, and Mirjana Sovilj
- *The Association for Prenatal and Perinatal Psychology and Health (APPPAH): BirthPsychology.com

Chapter 5: Creating A Death Plan

Resources for planning end-of-life care:
Books:
- *Dying Well: Peace and Possibilities at the End of Life* by Ira Byock, M.D.
- *What Matters Most: The Get Your Sh*t Together Guide to Wills, Money, Insurance, and Life's "What-Ifs"* by Chanel Reynolds (Note: Reynolds also has classes about how to get your affairs in order on her website, GetYourShitTogether.org)
- *The Art of Dying Well: A Practical Guide to a Good End of Life* by Katy Butler
- *Get It Together: Organize Your Records So Your Family Won't Have To* by Melanie Cullen & Shae Irving J.D.

Death Doulas or Death Midwives:
Some of these organizations offer, classes, end-of-life planning, and/or a certificate program for death doulas/midwives
- Going with Grace (Goingwithgrace.com)
- The Metta Institute (Mettainstitute.org)
- International End of Life Doula Association: (INELDA — Inelda.org)
- The Death Doula Collectives (Deathdoulas.com)
- The Death Midwife (Deathmidwife.org)
- Zen Caregiving Hospice Program (Zencaregiving.org)
- Doulagivers Institute™ (Doulagivers.com)

- Sacred Crossings: The Institute for Conscious Dying and Alternative Funeral Home (Sacredcrossings.com)
- Death With Dignity (Deathwithdignity.org)

Traditional Hospice & Funeral Resources:

- Hospice Foundation of America (Hospicefoundation.org)
- National Hospice and Palliative Care Organization (NHPCO.org)
- Hospice Care (Hospicecare.org)
- Funeral Wise (Funeralwise.com)

Green (Hybrid) Burial Options:

Each of these organizations, articles, and books offers a better understanding of what a Green Burial means and provides tools, guidance, and other resources on their websites.

- This is a list of green burial cemeteries in the United States and Canada: Nhfuneral.org
- Funeral Consumers Alliance (FCASMC.org)
- Green Burial Council (Greenburialcouncil.org)
- Natural Burial Association (Naturalburialassociation.ca)
- Natural Burial Company (Naturalburialcompany.com)
- Better Place Forests (Betterplaceforests.com)
- Aquamation Resomation (Aquamationinfo.com)
- Recompose (Recompose.life)
- *The Green Burial Guidebook: Everything You Need to Plan an Affordable, Environmentally Friendly Burial* by Elizabeth Fournier

I love the thought of my essence nourishing the trees. A wonderful reflection of this idea is best explained in Peter Wohllenben's book *The Hidden Life of Trees: What They Feel, How They*

Communicate – Discoveries from a Secret World, which highlights the interconnectedness with the forest's ecosystems.

*Music-Thanatology
Artists, Organizations, Podcasts & Books:

- *Music at the End of Life: Easing the Pain and Preparing the Passage* by Jennifer L. Hollis
- *From Behind the Harp: Music in End of Life Care* by Jane Franz, CM-th and Sandra LaForge, CM-th
- Roberts Music (Robertsmusic.net): Peter Roberts' recordings and books
- Threshold Choir (Thresholdchoir.org): The choir sings at the bedsides of the dying with chapters around the world
- Chalice of Repose Project (Chaliceofrepose.org): The Voice of Music-Thanatology

Videos, Podcasts & Meditations:

- Alua Arthur – A midwife talks about death planning – youtube.com – (search) Why I became a death doula (EndWell)
- Embracing End of Life by Patt Lind-Kyle MA (Pattlindkyle.com/meditations) – Guided meditations and exercises
- Mortality Minded with Thomas Gaudio (Mortalityminded.com)

Additional:
- Spirit Pieces Memorial Art (SpiritPieces.com)
- Titan Caskets (Titancasket.com) If you choose to bury traditionally, you don't have to buy a casket from a funeral home, this company offers more affordable options.

Chapter 9: Loss & Grief

Resources for all ages:
- Grateful Living (Gratefulness.org/light-a-candle): Light a virtual candle for your loved one
- Emotional Freedom Technique (EFT), a science-based exercise – TheTappingSolution.com or EFTUniverse.com
- Flower Essence Remedies – also see Chapter 3, "Making Friends with Death," for additional resources

For Children:
- The Dougy Center (Dougy.org)
- The National Alliance for Children's Grief (Childrengrieve.org)
- Emma's Place (Emmasplacesi.org)

Books:

- *Wherever You Are: My Love Will Find You* by Nancy Tillman
- *Lifetimes: The Beautiful Way to Explain Death to Children* by Bryan Mellonie and Robert Ingpen (ages: 3-6)
- *What's Heaven?* by Maria Shriver (ages: 3-6)
- *When Dinosaurs Die: A Guide to Understanding Death* by Laura Krasny Brown and Marc Brown (ages: 4-8)
- *Ida, Always* by Caron Levis and Charles Santoso (ages: 4-9)
- *Gorilla Thumps and Bear Hugs: A Tapping Solution Children's Story* by Alex Ortner and Erin Mariano (ages: 4-10)
- *I Miss You: A First Look at Death* by Pat Thomas (ages: 3-7)

For Adults:

- Grief Consultant/Author and educator, David Kessler (Grief.com): Offers free video series workshops and community support groups
- Grief Support Network (GriefSupportNet.org)
- Grief Recovery Institute (GriefRecoveryMethod.com): Offers a new view through The Grief Recovery Method

Books:
- *On Grief & Grieving: Finding the Meaning of Grief Through the Five Stages of Loss* by Elisabeth Kübler-Ross and David Kessler
- *Finding Meaning: The Sixth Stage of Grief* by David Kessler
- *Grief and Renewal: Finding Beauty and Balance in Loss* by Don Miguel Ruiz and Barbara Emrys
- *How to Live When a Loved One Dies: Healing Meditations for Grief and Loss* by Thich Nhat Hanh
- *The Year of Magical Thinking* by Joan Didion
- *The Grief Recovery Handbook, 20th Anniversary Expanded Edition* by John W. James and Russell Friedman
- *When Children Grieve: For Adults to Help Children Deal with Death, Divorce, Pet Loss, Moving, and Other Losses* by John W. James and Russell Friedman
- *Understanding Your Suicide Grief: Ten Essential Touchstones for Finding Hope and Healing Your Heart* by Alan D. Wolfelt (He also offers a journal companion book – sold separately)
- *Aftermath: Picking Up the Pieces After a Suicide* (Good Grief Series) by Gary Roe

- *How to Survive and Loss of a Pet: Comforting Tools and Practices to Embrace Your Grief and Heal Your Broken Heart* by Cheryl Richardson – Audible and CD available
- *Mindfulness and Grief: With Guided Meditations to Calm Your Mind and Restore Your Spirit* by Heather Stang

Chapter 10: Messages from Beyond

Resources:
Adult Books:

- *Visions, Trips, and Crowded Rooms: Who and What You See Before You Die* by David Kessler
- *Where Two Worlds Meet* by Janet Nohavec and Suzanne Giesemann
- *Proof of Heaven: A Neurosurgeon's Journey into the Afterlife* by Eben Alexander, M.D.
- *Bridging Two Realms: Learn to Communicate with Your Loved Ones on the Other Side* by John Holland
- *Communicating with Spirits: Meditative Methods to Help You Tap into Your Innate Medium Abilities* by Rita Berkowitz and Deb Baker
- *Reaching to Heaven: A Spiritual Journey Through Life and Death* by James Van Praagh

ABOUT THE AUTHOR

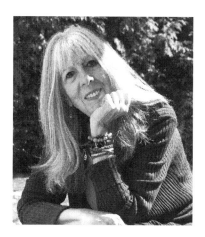

Kathy Arnos has been a pioneer in the field of sustainable living and holistic health since 1988. She is the founder of *Whole Planet Productions,* a health-conscious lifestyle hub — mind, body, and spirit — whose mission is to inspire, educate, uplift, and empower people to live their best lives fully awake, aware, and responsibly with a sense of connection to humanity and the earth.

Arnos began her professional writing career in 1988, by creating an in-print newsletter, *Mother to Mother: Another View, in* which she shared her daughter Danielle's personal story from poor health to recovery. The periodical transitioned to an online newsletter in 2006 as *Eco Family News* and ran until 2018, with a companion Internet radio show that she produced and hosted for three years on *I Am Healthy Radio.*

Arnos has served on numerous advisory boards as an expert, and authored two holistic parenting books, *Bach Flowers for Children: Raising Emotionally Healthy Children without Drugs (1991)* and *The Complete Teething Guide — From Birth to Adolescence (2004).* In the early 1990s, she produced and hosted a 30-minute show for public television, *Raising Healthy Children Without Drugs*. The *Los Angeles Times* dubbed Arnos "Medicine Mom," and *L.A. Weekly* called her the "Good Mother."

In 2005, Arnos created and produced a first-of-its-kind live event, the *Whole Children, Whole Planet Expo*, which premiered on *Earth Day* at the Los Angeles Convention Center and ran bi-annually from 2006-2010.

She has been featured in magazines and newspapers, appeared on national television and radio shows, and has been a contributing editor to various publications both in print and online for over 35 years.

In Arnos' latest book, *Walking A Friend Home: A Practical Guide to Consciously Living & Dying*, she addresses a deficiency in our society of the intimacy of relationships and offers readers tools, guidance, and resources to navigate the complex phase of midlife and beyond.

Walking A Friend Home represents Arnos' journey of the entire cycle of life — both in nature and our human experience, fostering love, balance, and respect throughout, eventually returning all elements to the earth. It reflects the importance of consciously living through all phases — including death. She weaves her knowledge, intuitive gifts, and connection to the spirit world together — facilitating gentle transitions full of grace, dignity, and a feeling of being loved with a sense of completeness for everyone.

You can connect with Kathy through her website at
www.kathyarnos.com